Peter Gordon is a sex therapist and counsellor working for the Family Planning Association. He has specialized in work on the personal counselling and training needs raised by the increasing incidence of AIDS and HIV.

Louise Mitchell is a clinical supervisor for the Diploma in Human Sexuality at St George's Hospital, London. She has wide experience of social work and now runs her own sex therapy practice.

some other titles in this series

Infertility
A Guide for Anxious Couples by Mary Anderson

The Menopause by Mary Anderson

Pregnancy After Thirty by Mary Anderson

Cervical Cancer
And How to Stop Worrying About It by Judith Harvey, Sue Mack and Julian Woolfson

The Dilemma of Abortion by Edwin Kenyon

Breastfeeding
How to Succeed by Derek Llewellyn-Jones

Everywoman
A Gynaecological Guide for Life by Derek Llewellyn-Jones

Herpes AIDS and other Sexually Transmitted Diseases by Derek Llewellyn-Jones

Preparing for Pregnancy by Philip Robarts

SAFER SEX

A New Look at Sexual Pleasure

Peter Gordon & Louise Mitchell

faber and faber
LONDON · BOSTON

First published in 1988
by Faber and Faber Limited
3 Queen Square London WC1N 3AU

Photoset by Parker Typesetting Service Leicester
Printed in Great Britain by
Richard Clay Ltd Bungay Suffolk

All rights reserved

© Peter Gordon and Louise Mitchell, 1988

This book is sold subject to the condition that it shall not, by way of
trade or otherwise, be lent, resold, hired out or otherwise circulated
without the publisher's prior consent in any form of binding or cover
other than that in which it is published and without a similar condition
including this condition being imposed on the subsequent purchaser.

British Library Cataloguing in Publication Data

Gordon, Peter
Safer sex: a new look at sexual pleasure.
1. Man. Sexual intercourse – Manuals
I. Title II. Mitchell, Louise
613.9'6
ISBN 0-571-15169-8

Contents

	List of Illustrations	vii
	Acknowledgements	ix
	Introduction	xiii
	List of Abbreviations	xvi
1.	Sexual Health	1
2.	Safer Sex in the Current Sexual Climate	18
3.	Taking Stock – A Sexual Inventory	30
4.	Back to Basics – You and Your Body	44
5.	Begining Again Alone	54
6.	Beginning Again with a Partner	72
7.	Safer Sexual Intercourse?	94
8.	Towards Safer Sex	109
	Conclusion – A Way Forward	126
	Appendix 1: Useful Organizations	128
	Appendix 2: Useful Addresses	131
	Appendix 3: Further Reading	135
	Index	139

List of Illustrations

FIG. 1 Female and Male sexual organs
       a) the vulva *page* 47
       b) The uncircumcised penis and scrotum;
       right the foreskin retracted 48
       c) The erect penis showing the glans penis
       and the frenulum 49
FIG. 2 How to use a condom 105

Acknowledgements

Several people helped to turn this book from a hazy idea into a concrete reality and we owe a debt of thanks to them all, including Esther Caplin whose inquiries prompted the idea, Bruce Hunter who gave us the encouragement we needed when we needed it, and Roger Osborne, Medical Editor at Faber and Faber, who recognizes a good idea when he sees one!

We owe a special thank you to Dr Elizabeth Stanley, who as well as teaching us most of what we know about sex therapy, kindly allowed us to borrow her 'ladder'. We accept full responsibility for the use we have made of this concept. We would also like to thank Anne Dickson for allowing us to use some of her ideas, in particular the Personal Inventory Exercise.

Toni Bellfield and Kaye Wellings willingly read the draft of this manuscript, at a time when they were both very busy with their own work, and made invaluable comments. We are very grateful to them both. Tuppy Owens and Meurig Horton supplied us with some useful details about organizations providing information on

HIV and AIDS and we thank them for their assistance.

We must acknowledge the contributions made to this book by our clients over the last few years in our different work settings. Even if they (or we) were unaware of it at the time, their trust and honesty enabled us to sharpen up our own thoughts and ideas about sexuality.

I also wish to thank Doreen who gave me the time I needed when I needed it. Last but never least, Hazel Slavin and Ewan Armstrong. Hazel made several useful comments about the text, offered suggestions for amending it, and when we needed it, challenged our assumptions and blindspots, and more important made me laugh! I'm glad to have her as my friend. Ewan not only read the book at each stage, but commented (as usual), offered suggestions and encouragement and, more important, taught me how to use the word processor! (Speaking of the word processor, thanks to Helen and that elastic card of hers, and to Paul Lewis for his timely intervention.) Additionally Ewan provided the material for the sections on HIV. Like many others I have benefited from his sensitivity and clarity of thought on this subject. Without him this book simply would not have happened.

Peter Gordon

I would like to thank the following people: Doug Linsell who has given me a few practical ideas and lots of encouragement and support; Ian Leslie, Linda Martin and Julianne Wight who have contributed some ideas and valuable criticism; Caroline Roberts; Francesca Bellis-Jones for ploughing through pages of longhand and converting them into something resembling the first stages of a book. Lastly, my deep appreciation to Peter Gordon without whom this book would never have been written.

Louise Mitchell

Introduction

This book is not about AIDS, but it is about the expression of sexuality in the era of AIDS and HIV infection. The fear of HIV (the virus which in some people may lead to AIDS) has brought many underlying sexual concerns to the surface. It is our contention that by addressing these concerns we can gain greater sexual fulfilment and avoid the dangers of infection.

Concern about the risk of HIV infection is justified, but this concern often becomes a vehicle for looking back at past sexual behaviour and worrying about the future. We cannot change the past but we can change our present and future sexual behaviour. In doing this we can discover more of our sexual selves, thereby increasing our enjoyment of sex and fulfilling our sexual potential.

Contrary to what we might have been led to believe, sex has never been entirely safe. Sex has, and always has had, a potential: a potential for pleasure, and also for pain whether physical or emotional. Sexually transmitted diseases, unwanted pregnancy, sexual abuse and exploitation are not new.

Safer Sex

While the principles of safer sex are relatively simple, there can be no guarantees about safer sex in the same way that there can be no guarantees about any other aspect of life. Sex is not something that simply happens to us; it is something about which we make decisions and choices. This book is about reconsidering these and about taking control of our lives generally in the light of one particular risk – HIV. Perhaps HIV and AIDS will finally give us the reason we need to reconsider our sexuality and what it means to us. This is also what this book is about.

Attempts to withhold or suppress information about sexuality have always been misguided. Telling us not to have sex may make some people feel better but it is not realistic. Instead of making scapegoats of those who, to date, have been most affected by HIV we should be addressing the difficulties and dilemmas they, and in turn all of us, may be faced with. People always have and always will have sex. Each of us is responsible for our own sexuality and how (if at all) we choose to express it, but in view of the potential risks attached to sexual activity, we need accurate information in order to make our own choices.

In many ways this book is as much about sexuality generally as about safer sex. We see safer sex as providing an opportunity to *expand* sexual and sensual horizons rather than limit them. As well as being good for your health, you might find that safer sex is good for your sex life, whatever your sexual preferences or situation.

In sex we draw upon and make use of the pleasurable potential of our minds and bodies. Therefore the more information we have at our disposal about our bodies and how to enjoy them the more effective we will be in appreciating them; also, the more able we will be to

Introduction

devise activities that are both sexual and safer. Feeling good about ourselves sexually can help us to feel good about ourselves generally.

What we hope to do is to give you the tools you need to decide what SAFER SEX means to you and how you can make the sex you have more safe. We are not going to give you advice. We want to offer you a way of finding your own answers to some of the questions that we all face.

We recognize that both safety and sex mean different things to each of us. What is sexually gratifying to one person may well disgust the next. In this book you may read words or see activities described which upset or disgust you. We are not advising you to do anything except think about the issues we are discussing. There is a wealth of sexual expression. You do not have to *like* what others do sexually, but you might learn to treat their sexual tastes with the respect with which you would like your own to be treated.

Similarly, safety means different things to each of us. One person's priority may be safety from HIV infection, while another's may be safety from pregnancy, and yet another's may be to protect herself or himself from abuse or exploitation.

Identifying what safe sex means to you is only the beginning. You need to find ways of expressing your needs for the kinds of safety and the kinds of sex you want. As a society we have never been very good at talking about sex. This affects each of us in different ways, so you will find that this book deals less with the mechanics of sexuality and more with the skills you may need to be able to deal with partners, to help you make the sex you have safer.

Safer Sex

List of abbreviations

AIDS   Acquired immune deficiency syndrome
HIV   Human immunodeficiency virus (the virus which in some people may eventually lead to AIDS)
STD   Sexually transmitted disease

1

Sexual Health

Safer sex – long overdue?

The current safer sex campaign was prompted by the gradual recognition of HIV infection, foreshadowed by the identification of AIDS. A safer sex campaign is long overdue given the large range of other sexually transmitted infections (such as gonorrhoea, syphilis, chlamydia). Why should HIV have prompted this amount of interest in safer sex?

HIV infection is potentially fatal and, as yet, incurable. However, other sexually transmitted diseases (STDs) have serious consequences, especially if not treated at an early stage, and some are still potentially life-threatening. Carcinoma of the uterine cervix (cervical cancer) is probably a sexually transmitted disease even if the actual cause is still disputed. However, HIV infection is unlike most other STDs in at least four important ways. First its incubation period is measured in years rather than days or weeks. Second infection is usually without symptoms for long periods, making it impossible to know who is and is not infected. Third most other STDs are easily recognized by men when *they* are infected: therefore men often go for treatment earlier (unless women are having regular check-ups). Finally unlike cervical cancer, HIV seems to affect men and women equally. Whatever the reasons, safer sex can enable us to enjoy our sex lives free from the fear of infection.

This chapter outlines some of the ways sex can be affected by the other aspects of our lives; from which STDs, including HIV infection, we can protect ourselves; and how we can use sexually transmitted disease clinics as part of a new approach to healthy sex lives.

Safer sex cannot be seen in isolation from the rest of our lives. We recognize that to be able to practise safer sex you may need to learn some new skills and have the opportunity to consider your relationships. (We provide a chance to do this in Chapter 6.) In this chapter we are going to look at some of the factors than can affect our sexual health.

Considering and practising safer sex takes time, energy and creativity. Contemplating safer sex may well mean considering those other aspects of our lives which affect our sexuality, for instance, health. A body which is punished by overwork, poor nutrition, too much alcohol, or insufficient relaxation, may well have little time or energy to contemplate safer sex.

You can keep yourself well and build up your body's ability to resist or control infection by following some basic guidelines. Most of these are concerned not with slavishly following fads and trends, but with assessing the degree of control you have over particular aspects of your life. It is important to do this as these may be adversely affecting your health and you may decide that some changes are desirable.

Diet

Good diet is a question of balance. Instead of simply cutting out various items from your diet, it is important to take a look at your diet and decide if it is sufficient for your needs. Do you eat regular meals or pick at snacks throughout the day? Are you getting enough roughage or are you regularly constipated? Is your diet very fatty and full of fried foods and salt? Do you ever eat fresh vegetables and fruit? Do you drink plenty of water? Do you look at the packaging on the food you buy to see what it is you are actually eating?

Alcohol

A little alcohol can have a very pleasurable effect on both your sexual feelings and emotional wellbeing. Some people find alcohol a powerful sexual turn-on and an aid to feeling more relaxed in social or intimate situations. Again it's a question of balance, of choice versus addiction. Are you drinking because you enjoy it or because you need it?

When it comes to safer sex alcohol can seriously interfere with your ability to make rational decisions. While we accept that it is often difficult to be rational when you are feeling randy, it does not help if you are also drunk. Alcohol may lead to a temporary carefree attitude, but the hangover the next day may seem nothing in comparison with the self-recrimination over not practising safer sex. A little alcohol can help you to relax in sexual situations but, more worryingly, it can interfere with your perception and judgement, with the result that you make decisions you may regret the following day.

The longer-term effects of alcohol can be as serious. Over a long period alcohol can affect our sexual health by interfering with sexual desire and functioning. It can affect our lives generally by becoming an addiction. Perhaps most important, as well as being physically dangerous if used long term, alcohol abuse can have disastrous consequences on personal, family and social relationships.

Tobacco

Smoking is linked to respiratory problems, lung cancer, heart disease, and contributes to the chances of women having a premature delivery or an underweight full-term baby. All of these are good reasons for not smoking, but as with any addiction it is not as easy as that. Addictions are seldom rational: they may meet needs, the existence of which we do not even recognize. It may be relatively easy to stop smoking, but the *desire* may well persist. There's no 'right' way to give up or cut down smoking. Smokers vary enormously in terms of what methods they have found most helpful to stop or cut down. A variety of books are now available on this subject, and if you are seriously considering stopping or reducing your habit it may be worth looking at a few of these. It is important to take things one day at a time, and to be kind to yourself, allowing yourself to have temporary setbacks and rewarding yourself when you feel you deserve it.

Drugs and their effects on sex

Many drugs interfere with sexual arousal. The effects of drugs are influenced by the dosage, the individual, personality, expectations, and of course the person's underlying physical condition. It may or may not make a difference if the drugs are prescribed, bought over the counter, used for medicinal purposes or recreationally.

The exact effect upon sexual functioning varies depending on the nature of the drug. Drugs can interfere with sex at various stages. Some affect desire, some the ability to respond (to get an erection or to lubricate), and some the ability to ejaculate or reach climax.

Oral contraceptives are often cited as causing depression, mood swings and decreased sexual interest; however, on the positive side, they may also decrease worry about pregnancy thereby diminishing sexual inhibitions.

Stress and strain

One person's stress is another's stimulation. This makes it impossible to make a list of particular stresses and possible ways of managing them. But it doesn't stop us recognizing and sharing how we each react to our own stresses.

For some the daily living routine may involve crowded polluted environments, using busy public transport or driving in traffic, meeting deadlines, juggling life around to fit in everything and everyone – this can be stressful – or it can be a real buzz! Sometimes it can be our own routines which are stressful and we might view the routines of others with envy.

For those looking for employment and or future career prospects, in need of adequate housing and enough money to live, it is little wonder that considerable amounts of time may be spent finding ways of getting by.

In short when we cannot realistically change the stressful situation itself, we can at least get by from one day to the next.

Safer Sex

People have recognized some commonly reported external stressors which put us under considerable strain: for example bereavement, the end of a relationship or marriage, losing a job and becoming unemployed, accidents, ill-health, examinations.

Stress can show itself in physical symptoms such as neck tension, headache and backache, skin rashes, stomach upset, insomnia. When we are stressed we seem more vulnerable to illness. Worrying about STDs and discussing safer sex may be stresses in themselves, but as with all stress it is important to pinpoint its source and make some relevant changes instead of struggling on hoping for the best or expecting the doctor to cure all your aches and pains.

Realizing that the effects of stress are showing can be a signal to slow down or make some changes. You may need to think about your lifestyle and reconsider what are the sources of stress in *your* life? What changes might you be able to make to reduce or get rid of these? Often all that is required is the ability to say 'no' to others, and to put your own needs first: finding the balance of work, rest and play in your life that is right for you.

Some of the most common strategies for dealing with stress are learning assertion skills (see Chapter 6), learning to recognize your own stress patterns as soon as they appear so you can deal with them, for example by having an early night or taking the phone off the hook. Many people find physical exercise a very efficient way of dealing with stress. This can vary from rigorous exercise like squash to more gentle activity such as yoga. If you decide this is for you, then choose an activity that appeals to you and give yourself time to develop your abilities.

If you are finding it difficult to manage the stress in your life you might look at some of the books available on the subject. Alternatively you might consider the idea of talking to a counsellor or therapist if you feel in need of support.

Finally, remember that nothing is unthinkable! If the situation causing you stress is unchangeable you may need to consider letting go and making more fundamental changes in your life.

The genital touch

As well as looking after your general health you can also pay attention to your sexual health by adopting some basic routines. These will help to keep your genitals healthy and less prone to infection.

It is important to keep your genitals clean. As well as helping to avoid infection this is also more appealing to partners. Uncircumcised men should draw back their foreskin and wash the penis to avoid the development of smegma, an unpleasant-smelling bacterial substance that can collect there. Daily washing with warm water and soap is sufficient. Chemical substances such as bubble bath or deodorant should *not* be used near the genitals as they can cause allergic reactions.

Making sure your hands are clean before touching the genitals, wiping front to back (from vagina to anus) for women, and using lots of soft toilet paper are simple measures you can adopt, as is the habit of washing your genitals and passing urine after intercourse or oral sex.

Some of the measures are more general such as: avoiding tight clothing since infections thrive in a warm wet environment; taking care of yourself when having a period, including getting rest if you need it and finding the tampon or towel that is right for you. Extra care is needed during pregnancy as it is a time of change for a woman's body and infections develop more easily.

Breast and genital self-examination

Breast cancer in women can be cured if it is identified and treated early enough. Similarly genital infections including cancer of the cervix can usually be cured if they are identified and treated early enough. So it is important to be familiar with the 'normal' state of your breasts and genitals. To do this you will need to become familiar with what they look and feel like, and to check them regularly for any changes. This involves paying attention to changes in appearance, feel, sensation, or the presence of any lumps or discharge. You should know your body better than anyone else and this might mean taking time to become your own expert. In Appendix 1 we suggest some sources of information to help you discover how to carry out your own breast and genital self-examination (see also Appendix 3: further reading). If you do have any concerns, act on them by going to see your general practitioner, well woman or sexually transmitted disease clinics (more on this later).

Genital examination is not only for women. Men can do this as well, recognizing any changes that occur, and acting on any indication that all is not well. Again, attention should be paid to any unusual change in appearance, feel, or the presence of any sores, lumps or discharge. Similarly, a useful source of information on this is provided in appendices 1 and 3.

Pelvic exercises

These exercises, designed to strengthen the pelvic muscles can be useful to both men and women. In women these can help to prevent or reduce the sagging of the internal organs, urinary incontinence, increase sexual responsiveness, enhance orgasm and prepare for childbirth.

In men, regular pelvic muscle exercise can strengthen the muscles surrounding the penis, help with erection difficulties and increase the intensity of pelvic sensation.

To do these exercises you begin by locating the pelvic muscles which you do by spreading the legs apart while urinating and stopping and starting the flow of urine. The ease with which you can do this tells you how strong these muscles are to begin with. The muscles you squeeze to stop the flow are your pelvic muscles. You can then exercise these muscles by alternately contracting for a second then letting go. You can do this ten times in a row then building up gradually to 15 or 20 or more. You do not have to be urinating to exercise them.

Since no one knows you are doing it you can practise this exercise anywhere, anytime, for example on the bus on your way to work, or while watching television. You can improve the tone of your muscles within several weeks.

Sexually transmitted infections

So far we have looked at some of the factors influencing our sexual health. It should be clear that all of us can learn more about our bodies and so take more control of what happens to them. This is nowhere more important than in relation to sexually transmitted infections, in particular HIV infection.

HUMAN IMMUNODEFICIENCY VIRUS (HIV)

It has been almost impossible to distinguish between what *is* known about HIV, how it is spread and how it affects people, and what has been *assumed* by newspaper editors, medical correspondents, television producers, health professionals and subsequently the general population. For many reasons, HIV infection has been exploited by many people to support their prejudices. This makes it difficult to establish what the current medical thinking is about HIV and in turn to make rational decisions about protecting ourselves and others whether or not we know ourselves to be infected already.

What do we know?
We know that HIV is very hard to catch. Realistically, for adults it can only be spread by very specific activities, namely

— *Unprotected penetrative vaginal or anal intercourse with an infected partner*

— *transfusing infected blood particularly through sharing infected needles and syringes*

For infection to occur the virus has to get from inside the body of one person to inside the body of another through the transfer of infected blood, semen or vaginal and cervical fluids. It is as simple as that.

A pregnant woman can transmit the virus to her unborn child, and there is also the risk of transmission through breast milk. But the actual degree of risk for any individual is unknown.

This virus is so fragile that it has *never* been shown to be transmitted through either social or sexual contact, which adheres to the principle 'on me not in me'! (see Chapters 7 and 8).

Sadly, the very specific ways in which HIV is transmitted have only become recognized over the last few years and before this many people became infected. We must all learn from this experience.

It might seem that a conscious effort is needed to put

Sexual Health

ourselves at risk of infection. We do have enough information to reduce our risk of infection while still living a satisfying social and sexual life.

What don't we know?
It is relatively simple to test blood for antibodies to HIV. It may appear to be commonsense to go along to a clinic for an HIV antibody test and have your worries relieved once and for all. However, what is still an area of uncertainty is the implication of a positive result to the antibody test. Most people who have become infected feel well and may be completely unaware that they have this virus unless their blood is tested. This test is *not*, therefore, an AIDS test, as it is so often misrepresented. A positive antibody result (often abbreviated to HIV ab+ve) suggests that a person has the virus, and is able to pass it on in the very specific ways mentioned already, *but* it does not mean that the person has AIDS. It does not even mean that the person will develop symptoms of the infection and become unwell. Acquired Immune Deficiency Syndrome simply means a list of signs and symptoms that are recognized to be the result of damage to the body's defences caused by HIV infection. At the moment, no one can predict who will become ill and who will remain well with this virus.

So what is the point of having the HIV antibody test? You might think that you have unwittingly put yourself at risk some time ago, or you believe that the information will help you adapt to safer sexual practice. Whatever the reasons, and after consideration some may be more rational than others, you must also consider what you would learn from a negative result as well as a positive one.

A negative HIV antibody result does not automatically mean that you are free from HIV infection.

Antibodies are produced by our bodies in response to infections, and the specific ones which are tested for to identify HIV sometimes take some weeks or months to be produced. Therefore it is possible to get a test result which means you are HIV antibody negative but have still been infected with the virus. If you think that you have put yourself at risk of infection recently, then a negative test result is not necessarily going to be a 'clean bill' of health.

Moreover, a negative result is only as reliable as it was on the day the blood sample was taken. If you have put yourself at risk of infection since your test, you might begin to ask yourself 'why did I have it in the first place?' Because of the implications of having this test, the uncertainty, possible discrimination, difficulties obtaining life assurance (to name but a few), it is essential that anyone considering having this test seeks appropriate counselling. This can be offered at an STD clinic.

A number of good books are available on HIV and AIDS, and some of these titles are given in Appendix 3.

OTHER STDs

We are all vulnerable to infections at some time in our lives, and anyone who is sexually active can get an infection which they can pass on to a partner with whom they are having sex.

Sexually transmitted infections are usually but not always spread by sexual contact. Many infections can be spread not only through sexual intercourse, vaginal or anal, but also through oral sex. Most of these infections can be treated but early diagnosis is usually important. The more quickly you detect the symptoms and go for help, the easier and quicker you will be treated.

Instead of listing all the signs and symptoms of all the

various infections we would recommend that you become familiar with genital self-examination (see Appendix 3 for suggested reading on this) and you pay particular attention to any of the following:

- unusual discharges or leakage from the vagina, penis or anus
- blisters or sores near the genitals
- rashes, itchiness or discomfort on or around the genitals
- greater frequency of passing urine
- pain on intercourse
- persisting lower abdominal pains

However, it is important to remember that you can quite commonly have an infection *without having any symptoms*, or symptoms not felt in the genitals. For example, with some infections such as syphilis or hepatitis the symptoms are more general, such as having a flu-like illness. Women with gonorrhoea or chlamydial infection often have no symptoms. Alternatively there may be internal symptoms which go unnoticed by you. You can prevent this worrying situation by making sure that you look after your sexual health by using the clinics specifically catering for sexually transmitted infections.

CERVICAL CANCER

Cervical cancer is the cause of thousands of deaths every year in British women – an appalling figure when we consider that these deaths are preventable.

Recent evidence suggests that cervical cancer may be caused by a virus which can be transmitted through unprotected vaginal intercourse. The human papilloma (genital wart) virus (HPV) seems to play a part, as does possibly the herpes virus. Other possible contributing factors include: smoking, sexual history of the partner(s), the use of oral contraception, the nature of sperm, smegma, chemicals, sexual activity, age of commencement of sexual activity, and pregnancies.

Needless to say safer sex has a major role to play in the primary prevention of cervical cancer whatever the cause turns out to be.

The majority of cases are cured and the disease stopped in its early stages. So why do women die? Some are embarrassed about or frightened of the smear test (the examination of a small scraping taken from the cervix with a spatula). Because of the hidden or unknown nature of the female genitals, and lack of sensitivity on the part of some health professionals, some women report that having a cervical smear can be an unpleasant or even traumatic experience.

Perhaps it is something to do with the status of women in this society that insufficient money and resources have been made available to invest in the prevention of cervical cancer. The number of people affected by AIDS in this country is so far small in comparison.

You can take steps to prevent cervical cancer by making sure that you have a regular smear test at your GP, Well Woman, Family Planning, or STD clinics. You should have one done at least every three to five years, more often if you are having abnormal bleeding or discharge. You may find the idea of having a smear frightening and therefore avoid it. The problem is that if you avoid having a smear, you are also depriving yourself of the benefit of early diagnosis and treatment of any potential problem. If you have never had a smear and are too frightened to do so you might consider ringing one of the agencies in Appendix 1 of this book and discussing your worries with them.

Sexual Health

You might consider using barrier methods of contraception or a condom for safer sex if preventing pregnancy is not an issue for you. Remember that cigarette-smoking may play a part in cervical cancer, so you might also think about changing your habit if you do smoke.

Regular smear tests are vital to protect yourself and are yours by right. A negative result indicates that no abnormality has been detected. An unclear or positive result means that you will need further tests. A positive result indicates the presence of abnormal cells. These can be destroyed without damage to the cervix if treatment is commenced at an early stage. If you are unsure what is being done to you *ask*, and keep on asking until you get a proper explanation.

USING YOUR STD CLINIC

These clinics are usually attached to main hospitals and are sometimes called special clinics, VD clinics or departments of genitourinary medicine. You can find out where your nearest one is by looking in the telephone directory under venereal disease, sexually transmitted disease, genitourinary clinic or special clinic.

The advantage of these clinics is that they are staffed by specialists with considerable expertise in their subject matter. They are free, confidential and anonymous. A letter of referral from your GP is not necessary and he/she will not be routinely informed of your results.

It is a good idea to ring the clinic and check when they are open and to ask whether or not you need an appointment. Remember that you do not have to think you have an infection to attend. If you are sexually active attending for regular check-ups is only commonsense.

The staff in these clinics are very experienced and

specially trained and will do all they can to help put you at ease. You may find yourself feeling embarrassed or uncomfortable at the thought of attending a clinic but remember that *everyone else is there for the same reasons.*

When you attend you will be given an appointment card with a number by which you will be identified from now on when you attend so it is important not to lose it. You will be seen first by the doctor who will take a history and carry out a physical examination. After this either the doctor or the nurse will take a urine sample, swabs and smears, and a blood test. You should never be tested for HIV without your consent. If you are in any doubt as to why particular tests are being conducted it is perfectly all right to ask. Women are examined internally and samples taken from the vagina and cervix. It is important to be honest when you answer the questions asked by the doctor about your sexual behaviour as this can help them decide which tests to carry out. It is highly unlikely you will be telling them anything they have not already heard.

It is sometimes possible for a diagnosis to be made immediately, and if this happens you will be given treatment there and then. More often, however, you will need to attend again for the results of your tests which can take a few weeks before they are available, and it is important that you do attend all follow-up appointments.

If you have an infection or have any specific questions you may be asked to see the health adviser who will help you consider how you will get your partner(s) to attend if this is necessary. This is important if you have an infection. You can be seen together if you wish. Even if the partner was a casual one he/she does need to be informed as he/she could have an infection without being aware of it, and may be passing it on to a current partner. Health advisers are able to provide information and emotional support concerning most aspects of STDs and sexual health and you can also ask to see her/him if you feel it would be helpful. They will also be able to answer questions you may have about the HIV antibody test.

If you do find that you have an infection you will be asked not to have sexual intercourse until this has completely cleared. You will also be given another appointment to attend the clinic to check that the infection has cleared. Annoying as this might be it can also be an opportunity to allow safer sex to start playing a part in your life!

Once you have been to an STD clinic a few times you will find that any fear you may have had should diminish. Clinic staff are usually friendly and supportive. It might help to see making use of your clinic as not only a right you have, but as a way of demonstrating your commitment to caring for yourself as a sexual person.

2

Safer Sex in the Current Sexual Climate

The current sexual climate is an unsettled and uncertain one, blowing alternately hot and cold breezes across the expression of our sexuality. We may have thought we were living in a time of great sexual enlightenment free of the taboos, ignorance and inhibition of yesteryear. However, increasingly serious sexually transmitted diseases, including HIV, are posing serious questions for each of us concerning our sexual behaviour, health and future.

The influence of the 1960s

Before we consider safer sex we need to understand something of the recent past and how it has influenced the current sexual climate. The 1960s were an important time in our social history. Legal reforms took place: of homosexual acts, of abortion, censorship and family planning. For those who wanted it, contraception, easier access to abortion, and a gradual relaxing of social attitudes made some forms of sexual expression more available. For those who believe that sexuality should be expressed only within a heterosexual marriage, the 1960s are looked on with horror as a time when the seeds of our present troubles were sown. For the radical the reforms of the 1960s mark the beginning of the sexual revolution, of a more democratic sexual morality.

Meanwhile, the media and advertising industries quickly realized that sex equalled profit and ruthlessly exploited sex for its commercial value. The images of sexuality portrayed exert a powerful influence on the way people think and feel about sex. Unfortunately this influence is often negative. The apparent new openness about sex was largely illusory as it was often based (and still is) upon titillating or romanticized images of sex.

The legacy of the so-called 'sexual revolution' is an encouragement to be sexually aware and active, to explore sexual relationships free from the fears of unwanted pregnancy. However, sex is still a focus for some people for ignorance and anxiety. The now added worry of increasingly dangerous sexually transmitted diseases is taking us even further away from the idea of sex as a potential source of pleasure and closeness.

Today's legacy

In the 1980s we are bombarded with images of sex leaping out at us from billboards, magazines, cinema and television screens. The message is that to be sexy we must be young, slim, attractive, wearing the right clothes and using the right shampoo. All these perfect young bodies on display can leave the rest of us only too well aware of our physical imperfections and feeling negative and inadequate about our bodies, particularly the more sexual parts.

Sex, we are led to believe, is what happens below the waist. 'Real sex' is two groins bumping away in mutual ecstasy. Much pornography reinforces this and presents the division of bodies into so many bits and pieces of sexual plumbing. You only have to fit the right bits together to achieve mutual delight, or so it would seem.

Little wonder then that some people have difficulty separating fantasy from reality – tabloid press nudes, wolf whistles, sexual harassment and rape are among the most alarming results of the way in which sex has become depersonalized and separated from the rest of our lives.

Sex education – a hit and miss affair?

These are some of the images of sex but what information do we get about it? It varies according to the country and culture in which we live, the school to which we go, the social and religious groups to which we are exposed, and the people with whom we mix. As therapists we spend a lot of time talking about sex with a wide variety of people, and we find that few of us hear much that is positive about sex. What we do hear is often inaccurate, misleading and frightening. This seems to be the case regardless of whether we are sixteen or sixty. We do not seem to have progressed very far.

Sex education is unfortunately also a heated political issue. The risk of HIV infection should be recognized as an opportunity to begin to get sex education right; to provide information about the range of human sexual experience, and an opportunity to clarify feelings, attitudes and values. It might also be an opportunity to present sex realistically in its social context, instead of on the basis of a hypocritical imposed morality. One political viewpoint regards sex education as corrupting young people and encouraging promiscuity. Proponents of this view regard it as a parent's duty and right to educate their children about sexual matters. This is in spite of the fact that a majority of both parents and teenagers have told researchers that they prefer sex education to occur within the school because of their discomfort in discussing the subject within the family.

If sex education is a hit and miss affair it does not seem to get any easier as we get older. Sex is a difficult subject to discuss. When mentioned it is often with embarrassed whispers, selfconscious dirty jokes, medical jargon or angry sexist language, usually associated with a good deal of anxiety and a painful struggle to find words which are not too rude, too vague or too clinical. Faced with all these difficulties we often avoid talking about sex even with partners. Rather than risk being seen as ignorant, unsure or pushy, we try to convince ourselves that sex does not need to be talked about.

The pressures of the 'sexual revolution'

Another result of the 'sexual revolution' is our endless preoccupation with sexual performance and success, often measured in terms of sexual mechanics and techniques. Speed of arousal, styles of 'foreplay', and whether or not intercourse and orgasm were 'achieved' introduce a rigid set of expectations and performance pressures.

Inability to live up to these expectations is a major cause of sexual disenchantment. For many people real or 'full' sex means intercourse. Anything less is not really sex, just 'foreplay' done in anticipation of the 'real thing'. The potential risks of sexual intercourse are becoming more apparent, but we have been taught that all sexual roads lead to intercourse: a suitably hard penis enters a moist and welcoming vagina, and after an appropriate period of thrusting both partners climax, preferably together and hopefully more than once.

For the sexually disenchanted help is near at hand or so it might seem. Glossy sex manuals, all claiming to help us become sexually skilled, adept or positively acrobatic, are constantly appearing; their popularity is a measure of the poverty of many sexual lives which value the permission of experts above their own innate creativity.

Deluged with images of sex the pressures to be sexually attractive and active are enormous and influence us from an early age. To say no to sexual intercourse at sixteen may be to risk being seen as odd, immature, frightened or frigid. At twenty-six or thirty-six similar pressures exist, even if we have worked out (at least in our heads) that we are entitled to say no. By sixty-six the pressure works the other way because we are led to believe that older people do not or should not have sexual feelings.

From the early teens we all experience the pressures to have a relationship in order that we can have our personal worth and sexual attractiveness recognized by someone and to be seen by the world as both desired and desirable. We live in a society in which being part of a couple is what matters. If you are uninvolved or celibate, you may find yourself having to justify your situation to other people and possibly even to yourself. Marital status is used to define and estimate us. Single people may be seen as somehow odd, inadequate, or just unlucky.

The range of choices

Today we are faced with choices other than marriage as the way to express our sexuality and meet our needs for intimacy – for example, living together, monogamy,

Safer Sex in the Current Sexual Climate

multiple relationships, open relationships and same sex friendships. Gay and lesbian relationships may be more visible than they were twenty years ago, but the speed and intensity of the way in which gay men are blamed for the HIV crisis reveals that *visibility* does not necessarily imply *acceptability*.

The range of choices may pose further problems. Getting what we want for ourselves from our sexual relationships rather than doing what we think society expects demands self-evaluation and self-confidence. Just as we were getting used to the luxury or perhaps burden of choice, the cold reality of HIV and cervical cancer emerges.

Long before the impact of HIV was recognized many individuals and 'movements' were challenging sexual stereotypes and conditioning. Some men were discovering that they could be gentle and nurturing, and some women were learning that ambition, assertion and independence were not necessarily male preserves. The feminist movement has changed attitudes dramatically towards sexual roles and behaviour, helping many women to explore and assert their sexual needs and desires instead of living up to the expectations of men.

For some of us sexual paradise may have seemed just around the next corner. Then we found ourselves in the middle of a crisis which seemed to sum up all the dilemmas and conflicts of the last twenty-five years. In January 1987 (six years after AIDS was first identified) it became official – 'Ignorance Can Kill'.

As we have seen already, 'normal' or 'full sex' in our society has been seen as sex that involved exchanging body fluids – penetrative sex – anal or vaginal. Having been used to this idea of sex we are now being told that this is 'high risk' sex and is possibly endangering our health. Red *'danger'* signals are now flashing where once

Safer Sex

the green lights encouraged us onwards in our quests for sexual pleasure. More anxiety and confusion! So perhaps it is no wonder that the concept of safer sex, far from being an easy panacea to all our worries about sexually transmitted diseases, is met with mixed feelings. What images come to mind when you think of safer sex – condoms, lubricants, rubber gloves, disease, a lifetime of celibacy, unnatural sexual acts? What feelings does safer sex evoke – boredom, disinterest, closeness, excitement, apathy, fun, frustration, fear of the unknown? Many of these are negative and perhaps this is because we are used to doing things, including making love, in particular ways and making changes in any area of life is seldom easy.

Relationships change, start and end. We have always found reasons for staying in relationships we may not really want. Fear of finding a new, compatible and 'safe' partner may be another reason to add to the list of finding a home, financial security, family pressure, the cat's welfare, as reasons for staying together. People who are in relationships now may not be in the future and may find themselves in a new situation where the concept of safer sex becomes a real issue in their lives.

Many people do not want to be in long term or short-term monogamous relationships. Suggesting monogamy as a solution to the risk of HIV is unrealistic, moralistic and inspires only reactions of panic, denial or avoidance. Monogamy may for some be morally safer sex. However, unless you know for a fact that neither you nor your partner is infected, and that neither of you *will become* infected, safer sex is something for you to consider.

For young people (or not so young, as people start sexual relationships at different ages) contemplating and wanting sexual relationships there is now an added

Safer Sex in the Current Sexual Climate

frightening and inhibiting element. Feelings about that first sexual experience can be very mixed – curiosity, nervousness, shame, fear of failure, relief or joy. The fear of sexually transmitted diseases can be an extra burden on what may be already an emotionally laden area.

Even for those who have had positive sexual experiences but are starting out again alone it is normal to feel nervous or apprehensive about getting involved again sexually and/or emotionally. It might be tempting to stay away completely (more about celibacy later) and avoid all the risks rather than face the possible dangers out there in the sexual jungle.

All sexually active people are potentially at risk which means that safer sex should be of concern to all those who care about their sexual health and pleasure. By now you may be thinking to yourself 'even if we accept in our heads that we might need to think about safer sex and perhaps even practise it (heaven forbid!) how could we actually enjoy it?' We hope that by reading further you may start to appreciate that as well as being good for your health, safer sex may broaden your sexual and sensual horizons and enhance the quality of your sexual pleasure and relationships.

We looked earlier at all the pressures on us to see intercourse as the normal way to make love. Sex is sometimes justified in terms of procreation rather than pleasure. Safer sex challenges us to consider this 'norm' carefully and begin to see the *whole* body rather than just the penis and vagina as sources of sexual/sensual pleasure, making us question our narrow focus on the activity (or lack of it) in our groins.

Negative images and feelings we may have about safer sex aside, other barriers may be preventing us from seeing safer sex in a positive light and making changes in our sexual activities.

Barriers to change

Here are some common responses to the idea of making such changes:

- *It's easier to stay with what I've got — I really can't be bothered.* Thinking about and practising safer sex takes time, energy and imagination.

- *Sex doesn't matter to me anyway.* Perhaps your sexuality is not an important or particularly rewarding part of your life so safer sex does not really rate as something to be considered.

- *I've just got my sex life all sorted out — not more problems!* Altering established patterns can leave us feeling vulnerable. It can be easier to stick to what we know.

- *I don't want to be different.* We have already looked at some of the pressures and expectations to have sex only in particular ways.

- *I wouldn't know how to talk about safer sex. What words would I use? — it's so embarrassing.* The facts alone are insufficient — many of us find it difficult to talk about sex, let alone safer sex, and few people feel confident in their communication skills to tackle this potentially difficult area.

- *What will my partner think of me?* If we do assert ourselves we may risk offending or scaring off a partner, or being thought of as aggressive, rigid, boring or a killjoy. We might even end up alone.

- *I don't have the right to ask. It's not up to me.* Your self-esteem and self-image may be low. You may not value yourself enough to believe you are worth caring about to make the effort. Safer sex is about respecting yourself and your partner, and taking control of and responsibility for your sexual expression.

- *It's all such doom and gloom* This feeling may foster 'a short life and a merry one' attitude. This may be all right if it is only you having the short life. What about your partner(s)? Failure to accept your responsibility may have serious consequences for others.

- *It doesn't affect me.* You may not be directly affected *now* (even if you could be sure) but you may be later. Considering safer sex now could be a valuable preparation for future relationships.

You can probably come up with your own barriers to change.

Making changes

In order to make changes in our sexual life (as in any part of our life) there has to be something positive to motivate us, some goodies that will make the difficult process of change worthwhile. Considering all the powerful barriers we have mentioned safer sex may not seem like a very appealing carrot.

It has been cultivated in a climate of fear, ignorance and punishment, heralded in as a pragmatic, easy solution to a complicated and distressing situation. We rarely like something when we are told we have to do it or because it is good for us. We ourselves have to accept in our heads and in our hearts that there *are* benefits and it is *right* for us as individuals.

So apart from preventing infection, what is in it for you if you practise safer sex? Consider that safer sex offers:

Safer Sex

1 An opportunity to be creative and imaginative and truly intimate in your sexual activities and relationships. You could end up broadening your sexual repertoire and increasing your sexual pleasure.
2 Safety from infection, conception and unwanted pregnancy.
3 An opportunity to break away from traditional sexual stereotypes – to do what feels good rather than what is expected.
4 An opportunity to explore the sensual and erotic potential of the whole body instead of focusing on the genitals. Safer sex can enrich and enliven a mundane repetitive sex life by emphasizing sensuality, affection, and communication and devoting to your sexuality the care, time and attention it deserves.
5 A way of taking good care of yourself – you are your own most important asset – deserving of caring and nurturing whether you are on your own or with a partner.
6 Encouragement to develop your assertion and communication skills in the area of sexuality. These can enable you to protect yourself from less obvious sexual risks such as abusive or unwanted sex, and can enhance the trust and intimacy within a sexual relationship. If you can talk about safer sex with your partner openly and confidently this may inspire you to tackle other areas of your relationship about which you are dissatisfied and wanting to change.

Strategies for change

Whatever your current situation safer sex could be meaningful and relevant to you. Whether you are without a partner and contentedly so, wanting to find a compatible partner, in a relationship and wanting to enrich it, or wanting to end a relationship and begin again, you may at some time need to consider safer sex. If you are confronted with the possibility of sexually transmitted infections then you will need to know how to deal with this in constructive ways.

In this book we present some strategies that may make safer sex more directly relevant and appealing.

First we begin with the individual and explore how we came to see sex in the ways we do. Having taken stock and understood where we are now, we can begin to assess what changes we may have to make to maintain a safe and enjoyable sexual life.

As individuals we need to be or become aware of and value our own bodies and sexuality first. We emphasize the importance of recognizing and developing all the senses since this enhances sexual pleasure and helps you to develop your own safer sex repertoire.

From the individual we move on to consider safer sex within relationships, looking at the assertion and communication skills needed to talk about safer sex with a partner. These skills can be learned and they provide the confidence to begin discussion and negotiation between partners to bring about the dual rewards of care-full and enjoyable safer sex.

3

Taking Stock – A Sexual Inventory

In Chapter 2 we looked at some of the more general influences on sexuality. We highlighted the pressure to conform and perform within particular acceptable limits.

We now want to identify and examine some specific influences, past and present, on sexual values and behaviour that affect us as individuals.

Taking stock helps us to identify misinformation, myths and taboos around sex, evaluate our current sexual lives, and decide what changes, if any, we might need to make.

Sex is a uniquely personal and individual experience. It is only by understanding how we come to see sex as we do that we can begin to get the information we want, and to acquire the skills we need to make sex safer and more pleasurable.

It is particularly important to recognize those influences that present sex in a negative, frightening or harmful way, as these can intrude into and spoil our sexual pleasure for the rest of our lives. As we grow older we may be able to dismiss early teaching intellectually, but on an emotional level we can still feel uncomfortable about certain sexual feelings or activities that we want to enjoy.

Even if you are not considering adopting safer sex it can be an interesting and illuminating exercise to carry out your own sexual inventory in order to appreciate more fully your own sexual attitudes, values and expectations.

What shapes the way we see sex?

The family

The earliest and perhaps the most powerful influence is that of our parents. What they teach us depends on their own learning, experience and comfort about sex. If they feel anxious, embarrassed or fearful then sex may well become a taboo subject within the family. If it is spoken about the messages may be negative and what is learned may leave us with the idea that sex is somehow unpleasant, shameful and certainly not a source of pleasure. Even if nothing is ever said we may still pick up the same negative feelings and ideas.

Other messages we may receive from our parents relate to our bodies. Some parents are able to encourage their children towards an awareness of and pleasure in their bodies and sexual development. However, many children learn that looking, exploring and touching are wrong or harmful. This is especially true for girls. There is often a general assumption that little boys will play with themselves because they are used to handling their genitals, but a girl's genitals are more hidden and can take on a more mysterious, unknown or forbidden element.

'Don't look', 'don't touch', 'don't enjoy' your body are very powerful negative messages that can stay with us even though in our heads we may have rejected them. Few people grow up believing that self-pleasuring or masturbation is a valuable way of learning about their bodies and an excellent preparation for later sexual relationships. In fact, masturbation is sometimes presented by parents as harmful to later sexual experience or as something childish, immature or perhaps even a necessary evil to put up with until one is in a relationship where real sex is intercourse.

A common myth is that only lonely, inadequate, single, undesirable, male people masturbate. Many people still do not acknowledge that women masturbate and enjoy it. Masturbation is seldom seen as a valid, enjoyable part of a sexual repertoire for one person, let alone something for two to share.

Because some parents may concentrate their attention and anxieties around genital activity in their children, even if we do hear anything from them it is likely to be about penises and vaginas. It is no wonder that our first ideas about sex are more to do with intercourse and babies and less about the whole body and other ways of being physically close. How we feel about touching and being touched may have its roots in our early childhood and family experiences. Our parents' and other adults' relationships are the first models we have. Perhaps they touched each other (and us) openly with warmth and affection; or perhaps they kept it behind closed doors as something private, associated with their lovemaking. Perhaps touch had aggressive or controlling implications and was used in an abusive way. As touch is such an integral part of safer sex it is important to consider what touch means to you – how and where and when you like to be touched.

The role of religion

What we learn from our parents and family about sex is often reinforced by the teachings of religions which value and desire the preservation of family life. Sexuality is presented within the framework of traditional heterosexual marriage and the nuclear family. High rates of divorce and the number of single parent families may be shaking the image of the nuclear family unit, but most religions refuse to accept anything other than monogamous marriage as an acceptable context for sexual expression. Vaginal intercourse (and the missionary position), because of its association with procreation is upheld as the mainstay of adult sexual relationships.

Many adults from strict religious backgrounds find that guilt and anxiety about masturbation, together with the emphasis on intercourse as the only acceptable form of sexual activity, are powerful inhibitors in their sexual pleasure. However, it is often not the religion *per se* that causes difficulties, but rather the ways in which particular orthodoxies or dogma as used by those who for their own reasons have an interest in suppressing freedom of expression in all its forms.

If the religion also forbids or discourages the use of contraception while simultaneously promoting intercourse, there may be additional burdens of risk, fear and resentment surrounding sexual activity.

Religions also shape sexual roles for men and women, often promoting a more passive homemaking wife and mother role for women and an active, providing, head-of-the-family role for men. There seems little permission, let alone time and energy, in this division for individuals to feel free to express their sexuality.

The role of education

As already noted, the current sex education debate in Britain means that many young people still do not get the chance to consider sexuality and personal relationships before these become realities in their lives. The quality of education about personal relationships and sexuality varies enormously, and is not helped by lack of sufficient resources for teacher training in this area.

Sex education may be provided within a biology and anatomy framework centring on conception, birth and parenthood. Again, vaginal intercourse is the focus of attention and presented as a goal to be achieved for sexually mature adults. Not much is taught about the whole body as a source of pleasure or other ways of sharing enjoyment and closeness. Of course, most of us older people did not even get the biology lesson, relying instead on the playground for our education about the facts of life.

Playground life has much to teach us about sex and relationships, but usually it is inaccurate, crude and derogatory towards gay men, lesbians, girls and women.

The differences between boys and girls emphasized within the family are reinforced within school. The sexes may be divided and this is reflected in the subjects and courses taken, employment opportunities, careers guidance and personal relationships. Boys are encouraged to be independent and achieve status through qualifications and financial success. For girls achievement and independence may be seen as incompatible with their traditional role. Such roles affect both how we see our sexual selves and how we behave. Boys are expected to initiate, to be knowledgeable and in control in their sexual relationships, while girls are supposed to be weak and compliant, ignorant and needing guidance

Taking Stock – A Sexual Inventory

by boys along the path to sexual fulfilment. Sexual experience is valued for boys and men and seen as normal and healthy. Although virginity in girls and women is no longer so much expected or prized it is still difficult for them to value their sexual desires and to be seen to be sexually active and initiating sexual relationships. These double standards which start in the playground with words like 'slag' and 'tart' for girls and 'superstud' for boys continue into adulthood. By the end of primary school many boys and girls will have at least seen the tabloid newspapers' images of sexuality, defining what is erotic and shaping their attitudes and expectations of sex.

At school we become acutely aware of ourselves in relation to our peers: what we look like, how we speak and behave become public matters. The pressure to be attractive, popular and sexually sophisticated can make school life a misery for some, resulting in a poor sense of personal worth and sexual self-esteem that can inhibit the later development of close adult relationships.

The role of the media

In Chapter 2 we looked at some of the images of sexuality in the media which pressure us to conform to certain ways of looking and behaving if we are to be sexually desirable. The media obsession with bodies (particularly women's breasts and legs) can leave those of us who do not fit the bill feeling negative and inadequate. For women, fears and fantasies about the size of breasts and buttocks, the amount of body hair and vaginal odour are mercilessly exploited by the advertising world and these anxieties can intrude into self-esteem and sexual pleasure. Although men's bodies are not commercially

Safer Sex

exploited to nearly the same degree, men also are affected by the 'perfect' image and can feel very concerned with their body size, strength and shape, particularly the size and appearance of the penis and testicles. No wonder it is so difficult for us to feel a sense of pleasure about our own bodies.

Some of the potential consequences of this might be:

– we might feel judged as a 'body', a collection of physical characteristics, not a whole person. This is particularly

Exercise: a sexual messages history*

> While reading this section you may have been reminded about things in your past and how they affect the extent to which you value yourself and express that sexuality.
>
> You may like to make a list of your answers to the following questions:
>
> – What were the first things you were told about sex?
> – Who told you?
> – How were they said?
> – What were the unspoken messages you received, even if nothing was said?
> – Think about the different influences in your life – parents, family, church, school, your peers, other groups or organizations you belonged to; think of what you read and saw in the world around you – consider all the current influences too. They all contribute to your present sexual make-up and how you choose to express yourself sexually.
> – Which of these messages have affected you positively/ negatively?
> – Which are still affecting you now?
> – Would you like to change any of these, if so which?
> – How might you do this?

*Adapted from Dickson (1985); see Appendix 3

Taking Stock – a Sexual Inventory

so for women whose bodies are often presented or exploited in relation to certain 'bits'
- we can feel a sense of competition with others
- we can be left thinking that we should be doing something to better ourselves
- we can start to resent our differences instead of valuing our uniqueness
- we might feel so inadequate that we just give up or abuse our bodies and ourselves
- we might become so self-conscious about our bodies that we cannot enjoy them

The realities in sexual experience

We have looked at the pressures on us to see intercourse as the only real or acceptable form of sex, but how does this relate to the reality of people's experience?

As sex therapists we spend time seeing people who feel somehow inadequate or sexual failures because they do not 'succeed' in penetrative sex or enjoy intercourse as much as they think they should, or because they prefer other sexual or sensual activities.

Men often feel they are under obligation to make their partner have an orgasm, preferably through intercourse, in order to feel sexually successful or before they can relax and enjoy themselves. This places pressure on them preventing their ability to relax and become aroused. Ironically this also contributes to problems in getting an erection.

The same pressures exist for women, who are similarly brought up to believe that intercourse is the ultimate experience of sexual pleasure. Some women, having invested the act with so many cherished hopes and desires, are left feeling 'is that it; is that what I've waited for'. Even if they and their partners appreciate the importance of clitoral stimulation and its role in arousal and orgasm, intercourse may be a disappointing and disillusioning experience. Recent research and studies indicate that although women may enjoy intercourse for a sense of emotional and physical intimacy, for many it is not the source of the most intense erotic pleasure and many women need more direct and prolonged stimulation of the clitoris for their sexual arousal and orgasm.

Difficulty with arousal and orgasm in intercourse is a major source of anxiety for some women, even if they are aroused or have orgasm with other forms of stimulation. Because intercourse is not the most rewarding of their sexual activities they feel sexually inadequate when this is essentially a normal female variation. Many women are now sharing their experiences, asserting their needs and challenging the emphasis on men's definitions of what should or should not be sexually satisfying, arguing instead that intercourse is one of a range of sexual options.

Some men too are also re-evaluating their sexual behaviour, realizing that they are not just a penis or some sort of sexual machine responsible for 'performing' for their partner. They too are appreciating that intercourse is but one way to share pleasure and closeness.

The problem of simultaneous orgasm in intercourse

This is yet another pressure to perform, and one more goal to be achieved if we are to be considered 'good at sex'. Some people define simultaneous orgasm as the ultimate in sexual harmony and 'success'. Of course it occurs and can be a source of great delight and intimacy, but if there is a pressure to attain it, enjoyment of each individual's pleasure may become difficult and even impossible as the whole experience may seem planned, engineered and controlled to ensure that one person does not get there first!

Sexual arousal and orgasm involves selfishness, self-indulgence and abandonment to your own sexual feelings. Part of your pleasure may come from seeing your partner's enjoyment, but if you are distracted by assessing your partner's degree of arousal, and trying to match your response to their's, your own mounting excitement and orgasm may be spoilt.

The ladder of sexual pleasure*

Sexual pleasure and sexual excitement can be enjoyed and shared at different levels of intensity, from cuddling to more erotic touching to orgasm, with or without intercourse.

To illustrate this we show sexual pleasure in the form of a 'ladder'; this presents it as something not geared towards performance, achievement and reaching goals, such as orgasm for an individual if alone, or orgasm for both through intercourse. Each step on the ladder can be valued and enjoyed for what it offers rather than as a means to an end. Individuals can experience different levels of pleasure on different occasions and likewise the intensity will vary for both partners each time they have sex together.

If you are with a partner, the performance pressure is usually greater. Sex cannot be divorced from an

*With kind permission of Dr Elizabeth Stanley

individual's moods, mental preoccupations and emotional state, or what is happening in the wider relationship. A couple is made up of two unique individuals and it is unrealistic to expect that both will be turned on or in the mood at the same time or aroused to the same degree. With a partner we can feel a pressure to be aroused so we will not let them down, but that may serve to make us anxious, which in turn can distract us from feeling turned on. This may prevent us from even getting to rung 1. Sometimes we just do not feel in the mood for sex – we may feel tired, sad or distracted by other events in our lives. Not to feel turned on does not mean there is something wrong with you or that you have failed your partner, it is just a matter of not feeling sensually or sexually inclined at a particular time.

THE LADDER OF SEXUAL PLEASURE

Rung 7	Good feelings after
Rung 6	Orgasm
Rung 5	Intense sexual arousal – discomfort if orgasm does not occur
Rung 4	Strong sexual arousal – full erection/lubrication
Rung 3	Moderate sexual arousal – partial erection/lubrication
Rung 2	Stronger physical pleasure – no genital sensation
Rung 1	Physical pleasure, e.g. cuddling – no genital sensation
Ground Level	No interest in physical contact or pleasure

STEPS ON THE LADDER

Ground level
This is the time when you do not even want to be touched or cuddled, for whatever reason. If, however, that reason is because of anger towards your lover which is left over from a recent or old conflict that has not been resolved then effective communication is needed. This means expressing your feelings at the time, not ignoring or repressing them hoping they will go away. They will not! They just simmer away and can intrude into letting yourself enjoy sexual intimacy.

We shall be looking at communications skills in more detail later.

Rung 1
At this level you may be feeling good physically and emotionally from touching or cuddling. It might be a more sensual experience naked than when clothed but either is pleasurable. A cuddle may be enough – you may not want any further intimacy.

Rung 2
This is the beginning of a more general sexual awareness. For a woman it may feel like an overall sense of wellbeing with more localized feelings of warmth or fullness in the genital area but as yet no vaginal lubrication. Similarly, a man at this stage may experience all-over stirrings of sensual pleasure with slight fullness in the penis.

Rung 3
At this stage there are significant physiological changes of sexual arousal and stronger sensual body feelings. The woman has sufficient lubrication and the man a

sufficient erection if they want to have comfortable intercourse.

Rung 4
The sexual feelings are stronger and more insistent but if you do not go on to orgasm you are not left with the physical and mental discomfort of 'being left just on the edge'. As with all the rungs this level is a valid sexual experience in itself and can afford considerable enjoyment without necessarily going any further up the ladder.

Rung 5
By this stage the need to have an orgasm is quite demanding and if you do not climax you may be left feeling frustrated and uncomfortable mentally and physically.

Rung 6
Each person's experience of orgasm is unique and each orgasm can feel different for any individual. There is a lot of pressure on people, particularly women, to attain the 'big O'. For women, orgasms have come to represent sexual self-awareness, liberation and success. Nowadays even one orgasm is insufficient as to be multiorgasmic is very much in vogue. Pleasure enjoyed at any other level on the ladder is somehow undervalued or totally negated by the emphasis on climax.

Rung 7
This is good feelings afterwards – the physical, mental and emotional satisfaction that may accompany an orgasm.

Taking Stock – A Sexual Inventory

You may like to compile your own ladder – with your own rungs that fit your sexual experiences. People, of course, do not necessarily go up the ladder the same way each time and sometimes it might be three rungs up, two rungs down! Neither do partners go up the ladder together and this is where problems may occur, leading to the importance of learning to talk about what is happening sexually and to negotiate and compromise in your sexual activities like any other area of your relationship.

For example, if one of you is at rung 5 and the other at ground level, then you might negotiate where you are sexually. One alternative may be for one of you to masturbate the other to orgasm with your fingers. You get your pleasure and your partner has not had to 'perform' for you, but has been able to enjoy the cuddle he/she wanted. There are no bad feelings here and you have shared a pleasurable experience. Both of you were able to get what you want without it being at your own, or each other's expense. But to be able to get what you want you need to have some idea of what is possible, so the next chapter looks at the physical possibilities – your body.

4

Back to Basics – You and Your Body

In Chapter 3 we looked at some of the influences on our sexuality. Bombarded by conflicting messages it can become difficult to sort out what feels good and pleasurable for us as individuals. Our own bodies may feel to us somehow disconnected and unfamiliar, possibly causing us feelings of anxiety, disinterest or shame. Safer sex might mean the need to change possible negative feelings into positive ones of pride, pleasure and respect. Safer sex means seeing your body as your own valuable property that needs nurturing and consideration, requiring time and energy, and deserving care and attention.

Safer sex is about becoming more aware of your body, developing your senses and becoming sexually creative.

Intercourse can be a way of limiting sensory enjoyment by concentrating on the genital area. It can also be a way of avoiding the intimacy that safer sex implies, as the latter means feeling, listening, looking, touching, smelling, exploring, which can leave us feeling more vulnerable and exposed than in intercourse. Some people experience intercourse as more anonymous and

Back to Basics – You and Your Body

an easy 'cop out' of feeling and being close. Safer sex may feel a threat because it confronts you with your feelings about your sensuality and sexuality and how you share this with a lover.

It is not too late to begin feeling good about your body – redressing the balance. A positive self-image means an enhancement of sexual pleasure and helps you feel more comfortable about safer sexual activities. If you are not worrying about your body and whether your partner is evaluating you then it is easier to relax and abandon yourself to pleasurable feelings.

Because we do not live up to certain ideals we may become totally self-critical or just ignore and dismiss our bodies as something not worth thinking about or caring for, or else just take them for granted.

When asked how they feel about their bodies, most people find it very easy to come up with a long list of criticisms and strong negative feelings. It is usually a much more difficult and self-conscious task to define positive aspects. We hope that our bodies will be appealing and give pleasure to our partners but we may not see them as attractive and valuable in their own right and take pleasure in them for ourselves.

EXERCISE: *personal body inventory**

In order to focus on your feelings about your body we suggest you take a body inventory. It is best to use a full length mirror and you will need a warm, private space with no distractions or interruptions.

Look at yourself in the mirror naked. Look all over from

---

*Adapted from Dickson (1985); see Appendix 3

Safer Sex

the top of your head to your toes – do not rush – try and spend at least ten minutes looking. As you look more closely at your body, ask yourself:

- What parts do you like most? Why? What do you like about them?
- Which parts do you like least? What is it that you do not like? How do you feel about touching them or having someone else touch them?
- Are you distracted by other voices criticizing your body? Some of the negative old influences you identified earlier may come to the forefront when you are looking at yourself. Try and concentrate on what you are thinking and feeling.
- How does it feel doing this exercise? Of what emotions are you aware – boredom, restlessness, curiosity, shame, interest, excitement, guilt, pleasure? What are your general feelings about your body? If you are a man do you feel you should be tall, broad chested and strongly built. Do you see your body as a machine to do your bidding? If you are a woman do you feel you should be a certain height and build – not too tall, too strong or too lean? Do you see your body as being to please others rather than yourself?

While looking, how aware are you of those parts of the body which are defined as more 'sexual'. Do you focus in on them very quickly, or are they the last parts you notice? Are they on your positive or negative list?

Often, those 'sexual bits' are the most difficult ones to feel good about – for women: breasts, buttocks, legs, vagina, labia (outer and inner), clitoral area; for men: penis, testicles, buttocks, chest. These can be laden with negative feelings of embarrassment, inadequacy, competition and failure.

If you have not spent time looking at those sexual

Back to Basics – You and Your Body

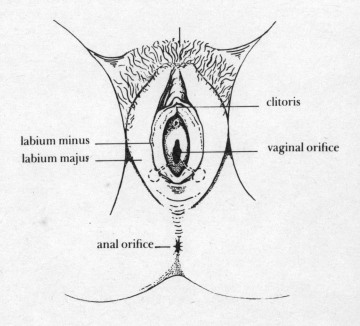

Fig 1a: The vulva

areas you might ponder for a moment on the reasons for this. What are your thoughts and feelings about these parts of your body? Have you always thought and felt this way? You might like to try the same inventory exercise concentrating on your genital area. It is important that you can come up with positive feelings about your genital area too and appreciate it as a valuable part of you which is worthy of your respect and care.

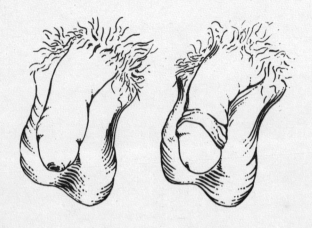

Fig 1b: The uncircumcised penis and scrotum;
right: the foreskin retracted

Getting to know our genital area

It is likely that some of us could describe our partner's genitals more fully than our own. We can take these precious parts of ourselves for granted or may become more aware of them if we are in a sexual relationships. Then we may be concerned that our partners will like what they see, touch, taste and smell and hope we are not too different or less attractive than what they have experienced before.

For those of us who got the 'sex is dirty' and 'you don't touch down there' message, the fear of sexually transmitted diseases can make the genitals seem even more

Back to Basics – You and Your Body

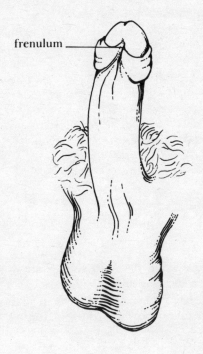

Fig 1c: The erect penis showing the glans penis and the frenulum

like danger zones to be avoided.

Looking closely at your genitals may feel like a strange, silly or indulgent thing to do. You may feel anxious about what you will discover, and the thoughts and feelings that may emerge which have been influenced by what you have seen, learnt and experienced during the course of your life; much of this might be negative. Think of where the negative feelings come from, then try and focus on the positive ones. You may need to look on several occasions before you feel comfortable and can appreciate the uniqueness and attractiveness of your genital area. If you feel comfortable with looking at and touching this area of your body, along with all the other parts, you will be well on your way to devising and enjoying your own safer sex. Familiarizing and valuing your genitals as a precious part of you is an important part of your enjoyment of your own sexuality and even more important now as you are considering what safer sex means to you.

Sexual language

Consider what you call the different parts of your genital area.

If you are a woman it is often very difficult to find words which feel right, particularly as some words are used in such a derogatory or aggressive way against women. Words like vagina, clitoris, labia, penis, testicles, foreskin may feel too clinical or formal, but others like cunt, pussy, cock, prick, balls may not appeal to you either. Expressions like 'down there' or 'between my legs' do not help much because of their vagueness. Later we demonstrate some of the words which describe sexuality, but it is possible that you will find there are only a few that are acceptable to you. If you do not like them, you can always make up your own words. But if you do not feel that creative, think about the words you already know and what it is about them you dislike. Do they sound rude? Are they too sexy? Is it foul language for you? Is it politically offensive? Do they turn you on? Would your mother be shocked if she heard you use them? Words can be sexually arousing and give us

Back to Basics – You and Your Body

pleasure but there can be barriers to using them to enhance our sexual experiences. Again, these barriers can be related to past learning and experiences. However, words are *safe* – they are yours to use and enjoy.

Often we rely on extrasensory perception or guesswork in our sexual communications, hoping that our partners will touch the right part of our body in the way we like. However it does not necessarily work out that way. If we have words and use them we can help ourselves and our partners to eliminate the guesswork that can cause fatigue, frustration and resentment on both sides. Talking about sex does not mean that sensitivity, spontaneity and imagination are sacrificed along the way. It just means more effective communication and enhanced pleasure.

If you are going to enjoy safer sex looking and being comfortable with your body is a very positive beginning. If you have done the exercises already mentioned (page 45), hopefully you will have begun to appreciate your body as your own valuable property. The whole body offers opportunities for sensual pleasure either alone or with a partner. Just looking at our own body and/or our partner's body can be very pleasurable without necessarily leading on to more erotic content (remember the different rungs on the ladder).

Self-pleasuring exercise

Of course it was not always like this. As babies we took delight in our bodies and their natural functions. Most of us on the way to adulthood lost our innocent sense of innate sensuality, and learned to become 'disconnected' from our bodies. This next exercise is about trying to remake that connection.

Having spent some time looking at and rediscovering your body, you may like to move on to a self-pleasuring exercise. Self-pleasuring may seem a strange concept at first. It may feel selfish, self-indulgent, a waste of time. A lot of us grow up with the idea that giving to ourselves is harmful or wrong or immature and that somehow 'to give is better than to receive'. That often applies to sex too. Some people believe that they must take care of their partner's pleasure first before they can enjoy their own or that if they get any pleasure for themselves that is a bonus but not necessarily important. Taking pleasure for yourself is just as important as giving it. Safer sex can be a challenge to your idea of sexual pleasure by encouraging you to find out what is pleasing to you rather than going along with established patterns.

This self-pleasuring exercise involves developing sensory awareness of your whole body. Our *brains* are the most important sex organs we have. We have many different senses – sight, smell, taste, hearing, touching – and developing these senses can enhance sexual enjoyment and be enjoyed safely (more on this in Chapter 8).

EXERCISE: *Self-pleasuring*

We would suggest you spend thirty minutes on the following self-pleasuring exercise. Make sure you have privacy and will be free from distractions.

– Take time to create a relaxing, sensual atmosphere using whatever stimuli you like. Remember this is for you – you do not have to please anyone else. You may like mirrors, music, candlelight, incense, a glass of wine, your favourite pictures around you. Use your imagination.
– You may like to start with a relaxing bath or shower

Back to Basics – You and Your Body

where you can pamper yourself. Enjoy the soothing effects of the water against your skin or the pleasure of soaping or just touching your body.
– Using a body lotion, oil or powder, if you prefer, give yourself a light massage all over. Focus in on the different physical sensations you feel in different parts of your body; notice the different skin textures and muscle tone. Be aware of the pressure of your touch – do some areas respond more to a lighter or firmer touch?
– You may discover places you have not touched before. Explore them. It may be very pleasing to touch or stroke new areas. Give yourself permission to enjoy your body.

This self-pleasuring is not designed to turn you on but it may do – if so, just *feel* the sensations, do not try and increase them. You do not have to perform or please anyone else. There is no hurry here and there are no demands on you.

If you feel comfortable with your body and know how and where you like to be touched, this will help increase your awareness of your sensuality and hence your sexual pleasure. Also, if you know what it is you like you will then be in a better position to talk to a partner about sex. Irrespective of whether you are in a sexual relationship or not you are still a sexual person in your own right. To learn about your body and know what pleases you are important aspects of appreciating your own sexuality.

In the next chapter we will be looking at being safely and enjoyably sexually active – alone.

5

Beginning Again Alone

One of the most powerful lessons we learn about sex is that it is something we do with other people. Being sexually active implies that you have a sexual partner and are sharing sexual activities, hopefully to your mutual satisfaction. Having a sexual partner is viewed as the normal and desired relationship status in our society. The image of the 'couple' is all-pervasive and the pressures on all of us to have a partner encroach upon us at every turn. We are not suggesting that to desire and enjoy a sexual relationship is only a response to social pressures. For many people a close relationship offering sexual pleasure is an important part of life and should be respected as a valid choice. However, because there is so much pressure to be in a sexual relationship we forget that we are sexual creatures in our own right, capable of experiencing a range of sensory pleasure *alone*. We would suggest that celibacy is not synonymous with sexlessness or lack of sexual activity. Even though you are not having a sexual relationship you may still respond sexually and actively to sensual and erotic stimuli. You may still have sexual thoughts, dreams, hopes, fantasies, feelings, desires, through which you are expressing your sexuality. Just by being you – the way you look, speak, act and relate to others is a reflection of your sexuality.

Celibacy and you

The word celibacy itself sounds cold and harsh and may conjure up negative feelings and images. It is often the first thing that comes to mind when people think of 'safer sex' and along with it may be associated fears and anxieties of being alone for a while, possibly a lot longer than you would like. Celibacy may feel all right for a while but the thought of it going on and on may be very uncomfortable, depressing and even frightening.

Think of what celibacy means to you. Perhaps you are celibate now or are contemplating the end of a relationship soon. Perhaps you have always gone from one relationship to another and have had no time on your own out of a sexual relationship. Maybe you have not had a sexual relationship yet and are very eager to find a partner.

Perhaps you are in a relationship that was once sexual but now is not, possibly because of unresolved personal or relationship difficulties that have intruded into the sexual side of the relationship.

When asked about feelings and attitudes towards celibacy most people respond negatively. Consider the following:

– Everyone else is in a relationship and I feel like I'm missing out.
– I don't feel attractive – I need someone else to tell me they fancy me.

Safer Sex

- I'll forget how to do 'it' – it'll be so difficult starting again.
- My friends don't ask me over because they are all in couples and I'm not.
- I'm losing my confidence and don't want to go out alone.
- I'm scared that I'll look desperate for a relationship and frighten possible partners away.
- It might be safer sex but it's boring!
- People think I'm strange or feel sorry for me.
- I feel there must be something wrong with me – it seems so easy for everyone else.

These feelings can be very strong and damaging to your self-esteem just when you might be feeling low or vulnerable anyway. We are not trying to dismiss the validity of these feelings, but if we look closely at them we may be able to trace them to some commonly held myths in our society about celibacy.

MYTHS ABOUT CELIBACY

Celibate people are:

- unattractive, undesirable and not valued
- lonely, isolated and deserving of sympathy
- at best somehow odd, at worst pathological
- undersexed or not interested in sex otherwise they would not put up with it
- sexually frustrated, perhaps desperate for sex and therefore not very discriminating
- deficient emotionally, for example, cold or unfeeling and not a good proposition for a relationship

- harmed physically or emotionally
- not leading a full life because they are not expressing their sexuality in a relationship
- selfish, demanding, used to taking care of themselves, finding it difficult adapting to a give and take emotional/sexual relationship
- sexually inadequate or poor lovers otherwise they would be in a relationship
- more likely to commit sexual offences or engage in deviant acts because they have no outlet for their sexual expression.

With all these myths around no wonder it is hard to have any positive thoughts or feelings about celibacy and value it as an acceptable sexual alternative.

POSITIVE ASPECTS OF CELIBACY

So apart from being the best protection from sexually transmitted diseases what are the positive aspects of celibacy?

- Celibacy can be a constructive period of 'time out' providing an opportunity to think about what you want from a sexual/emotional relationship without the pressures of being in one.
- Sexual relationships take time and energy – you can put these into developing other relationships which you value or into other activities which you enjoy or are demanding of your physical and/or mental energy.
- Celibacy can confront us with our sexual needs and desires; it can be a valuable time for learning about and defining what is pleasurable for us.

- Sex is not the only way to meet our needs for physical warmth and affection. Sometimes the first is traded in order to get the latter. Celibacy prompts us to find other ways to find some of the physical nurturing, touching and affection we may be seeking.
- Celibacy can be a time to care for yourself. It may even be part of a healing process, for example, if you have just finished a relationship or may be grieving or depressed you may need time just to be by yourself.
- A learning process about being alone and testing out your independence and discovering what it means to you. Being on your own comfortably can be a very valuable life skill because when you do enter a relationship it will be through choice rather than through fears of being alone.
- Celibacy means you do not have to concern yourself with another person's sexual needs which means you can think more about you and your pleasure. This is a constructive selfishness – many of us learn very early that we have to put others' needs before our own and take care of others first.

You might think about what celibacy means to you. Do you see it as a bore, a prison sentence, a deadening of your sexuality, or do you see it as a challenge, a time for stocktaking and learning and another way of expressing your sexuality? If you are celibate, is it your choice, due to fear of disease? If so you may need to look at your fears and get some accurate information to help you make some decisions about your life. As we have said, celibacy does not mean the end of your sexual desires or needs. These go on and need to be expressed and satisfied. Many people find this outlet through masturbation but for some this is associated with guilt and anxiety.

Masturbation

Masturbation is still a taboo subject and riddled with a host of negative associations. That is why some people refuse to consider it as simply an item on the sexual menu. They would prefer not to masturbate at all and wait until the next sexual partner comes along. This is more true of women for whom the inhibitions to masturbate are greater, probably because of cultural conditioning. Generally, women are not encouraged to be sexually self-sufficient and feel good about taking their own pleasure for themselves. They may learn to wait until a man comes along who will then open their eyes to the wonders of sex and lead them down the path to sexual fulfilment through heterosexual intercourse. Women may enter sexual relationships lacking knowledge, confidence and a sense of sexual independence.

Men appear to masturbate more readily than women but few view it in a very positive light. Their cultural conditioning leads then to equate sexual success with being sexually active with a partner. Being alone and 'having to' masturbate is for many a powerful assault on sexual self-esteem.

We believe that masturbation is, apart from being very safe sex, a very important part of each individual's sexuality. On the journey to sexual enlightenment and pleasure we would advocate it as being the first stop and a vital base for feeling knowledgeable, confident and secure in our sexuality. Let us look at some of the common myths about masturbation which affect our views.

Safer Sex

MYTHS ABOUT MASTURBATION

It is 'infantile' sexuality to be abandoned on adult maturity.

- It is a poor substitute for 'the real thing', that is intercourse.
- It takes over and becomes compulsive – once you start you cannot stop.
- The desire to self-pleasure stops when you are in a relationship.
- It is harmful: physically/mentally/emotionally.
- Orgasms from masturbation are inferior to those in other lovemaking.
- Masturbation is a private thing, to be done alone, not shared.
- Sex is for giving to someone else, therefore masturbation is selfish and self-indulgent.
- Only lonely, isolated, inadequate people masturbate.
- Men masturbate but women do not want to or need to.
- Getting used to having orgasms through masturbation stops you being able to have them with a partner.

As with the myths about celibacy, those about masturbation are quite powerful and negative and can be strong inhibitors to our sexual self-esteem and enjoyment. We may reject the myths, the taboos and the 'don'ts' about masturbation, but we may still feel anxious, uncomfortable or guilty about it. The word itself, like celibacy, sounds formal and clinical and a long way off from anything to do with pleasure. The many slang words for masturbation are mostly male terms, for example jerking off, wanking, self-abuse, associating it with something mechanical, pleasureless or even harmful. Because of the taboo nature of the subject the words may be used

Beginning Again Alone

jokingly or scornfully. You might have your own positive word(s) for it that suit you. We sometimes use the phrase self-pleasuring (remember back to the self-pleasuring exercise in Chapter 4) to include genital self-stimulation, that is, masturbation, whether it be at a low level of sensory pleasure or anywhere along the ladder of sexual excitement including orgasm.

Having looked at some of the myths about masturbation let us look at some of the positive aspects of this much maligned and underrated sexual activity.

POSITIVE ASPECTS OF MASTURBATION

The following are some of the good things about masturbation:

- It is an act of rediscovery; little children take an active pleasure in self-exploration and touching, only later do they become self-conscious about it.
- We learn about our own eroticism – what we like and need for ourselves as individuals; we are unique and can become our own experts.
- We learn to value our genitals and enjoy our own arousal and/or our own orgasms.
- It is good for you! Masturbation keeps your sexual equipment in good working order. For women it keeps the vagina lubricating and helps to maintain a healthy vaginal environment. Some women find that an orgasm can help alleviate period cramps and pelvic congestion. For men, masturbation keeps the erection and ejaculation reflexes working.
- It is a valuable way of being sexually independent, and an excellent preparation for later sexual relationships. If both partners each take individual responsibility for meeting their own sexual needs sometimes

and enjoy masturbation as another item on the sexual menu, then this both enriches the sexual repertoire and relieves the burden of expecting our partner to always equal our level of desire or meet our sexual needs. If you know what you like you can teach your partner, which saves a lot of guesswork, discomfort and frustration.

- For women who have not experienced orgasm, masturbation can provide the intensity of sexual stimulation away from any pressures to 'perform' with a partner that is necessary to have an orgasm. It may be difficult for some women to get to this stage if they have negative feelings about giving pleasure to themselves but it is well worth putting some time and energy into this self-discovery.

- Masturbation is an abandonment to your own pleasure – it is loving yourself, being self-indulgent, letting yourself go physically, mentally and emotionally. It helps you to relax and relieve sexual, physiological and psychological tensions.

- It is legal, non-fattening, safe and always available.

- We do not know when we may be on our own. If we can enjoy our own sexuality and achieve some degree of sexual independence and confidence, then we are in a better position to make a discriminating choice in our next sexual partner and not rush into an unsatisfying relationship through desperation or sexual frustration.

- The degree of physical pleasure derived from masturbation, from arousal through to orgasm, may be just as intense or even more so than that experienced in other sexual activity.

SELF-PLEASURING

Before we go on to look at some of the many and varied ways that women and men self-pleasure, we would like to make a few points about self-pleasuring which are important if you are going to get the most enjoyment you can from it.

- Self-pleasuring, like any sexual activity, requires time, energy and a little imagination. If it is rushed or too repetitive, or done when you are tired or preoccupied with other things, your desire to self-pleasure or the enjoyment obtained may be reduced.

- How you feel about self-pleasuring will affect the quality of the enjoyment. If you feel anxious or guilty about it try and identify where those feelings come from – perhaps they are linked to some of the myths already mentioned or perhaps they are related to early negative teachings or experiences. Think about what self-pleasuring means to you – read books about it (see Appendix 3). Hopefully then you can put a few ghosts to rest and give yourself permission to enjoy yourself.

- Self-pleasuring, like lovemaking, can become a very genitally focused activity. If you tried the earlier exercise about pleasuring your whole body you will appreciate that the latter offers opportunities for sensual and erotic pleasure. Hopefully by now you will have discovered where and how you like to be touched and you can include this with more erotic genital stimulation when you are self-pleasuring.

- Remember that you have other senses besides that of touch and these can be developed and used to enhance your self-pleasuring.

- You may not always feel like creating a special atmosphere each time, but do not neglect those other senses:

smell – try perfumes, lotions, incense, natural body odours, food, cooking smells, etc.; taste – food, drink (not too much as this may dull other sensory awareness), skin taste, body secretions, etc.; sight – looking at yourself while you are pleasuring, using mirrors, reading erotic material or looking at pictures that you find arousing.

– Imagination: think about sexy things that you have done in the past or would like to do. Create your own sexual fantasies. This might be difficult at first if you have not tried it before but if you practise it just by starting off with a few thoughts or pictures in your mind you can develop the images in time. It might help to read about other people's fantasies (see Appendix 3) just to give you a few ideas. Many people use fantasy to enhance their self-pleasuring – it is normal, safe and just another expression of your sexuality. Fantasizing can be a very useful way of focusing in on your sexual feelings and building up your excitement, particularly if you find yourself distracted by other intrusive thoughts or feelings. People fantasize about all sorts of situations. What is a turn on for some may be a major turn off for others. Do not worry about the content – it is just your sexual imagination working overtime for your enjoyment and they *are* only fantasies, and not going to be acted on in real life. Fantasies are private and *you* are in control. If, however, you feel *very* uncomfortable about the themes or content of particular fantasies you could try and tone them down or alter them to find others which are more compatible with your values but are pleasurable nevertheless.

We shall be looking in more detail at using all the senses when we talk about the practicalities of safer sex.

Beginning Again Alone

Just to give you a few ideas we are going to look at some of the more common techniques of self-pleasuring for women and men. We are not telling you that you should be self-pleasuring in any particular way – you will decide what you like and what is best for you.

You may like to consider some of the following.

TECHNIQUES OF FEMALE MASTURBATION

Hand techniques
Using one or more fingers or the whole hand. You might start gently, caressing the whole genital area then moving gradually to more specific areas, such as outer or inner vaginal lips, inside the vagina, the clitoris. The clitoris is very sensitive – if you stimulate there too quickly or harshly you may experience discomfort; – if so, move away and build up your arousal before returning to the clitoris or be very gentle to start with and gradually increase clitoral stimulation. You can vary your movements, going in circles or caressing up and down, as you like – you can alter the speed depending on what feels good.

Many women find touching their anal area can be very pleasurable – if a finger (or any other safe object, such as a vibrator) is inserted into the anus then care should be taken to wash the finger or object before any penetration into the vagina, as bacteria can easily be passed leading to vaginal infections.

Your breasts and nipples are very sensitive to touch and may give you much pleasure. Experiment with different ways of touching, caressing and squeezing. You may play with breast(s) and nipple(s) with one hand, leaving your other hand free to pleasure your genitals.

You can try different positions – lying on your back,

side or stomach; sitting, standing, crouching – use your imagination.

We are all voyeurs to a certain extent, and watching yourself while you self-pleasure may be as big a turn on as looking at a partner, or sexually explicit photos or movies. If you have a mirror you might try pleasuring yourself in front of it. You may be naked or partially clothed.

Do not forget your pubic hair – brushing your hand against it or caressing or gently tugging it can be quite sensual.

An extrasensory bonus to hand techniques can be the use of lotions or oils. But use something without chemical colorants or perfumes as this may cause irritation.

Other techniques
Apart from your hands you may use other objects which may help your self-pleasuring. Here are just a few:

- A pillow placed between the legs when lying face down. Holding legs quite firmly and pressing pillow against the clitoral area. You can also try this with a hot water bottle but be careful that it is not uncomfortably hot.
- Water pressure from the shower hose or from the bath taps, letting the water go directly onto the genital area.
- Pressing the genital area against some vibrating object, such as a washing machine.
- Some women derive sexual pleasure from pressing their thighs together and alternating between contracting and relaxing their pelvic muscles.

Vibrators are becoming more and more popular as

Beginning Again Alone

sexual toys, affording their users an extra dimension of sexual pleasure. Some women who have been unable to climax with a partner or with other self-pleasuring techniques find they are orgasmic with a little help from a vibrator. Vibrators can give quite a powerful and consistent sexual stimulation which some women need to become aroused and climax. Their advantage is that they keep on going and you are at the controls. You can pleasure yourself all over with the vibrator and use your free hand to stimulate other areas of your body while your vibrator is focusing on another. As with using your hand, direct stimulation of the clitoral area with a vibrator may cause discomfort – you may like to leave your pants and/or trousers on and feel the vibrations through the cloth, or otherwise wrap the vibrator in some soft sensuous material which provides an added bonus to pleasure.

Some women feel initially hesitant or negative about using a vibrator: 'it's mechanical – it can't be right making love with a machine', 'I might always need it to get aroused – what will I do when I'm in a relationship' or 'I shouldn't need it – it's not real sex anyway'.

Try and see it as just another way of giving yourself pleasure safely. It will not take over your life, or interfere with forming a later sexual relationship – chances are that it will enhance it as you are capable of taking care of your sexual needs and have added another safe and enjoyable item to your sexual repertoire which you can if you choose share with your next partner. They will probably find it a turn on too and you can experiment with using it in your love-making. We shall be talking more about vibrators in Chapter 8.

TECHNIQUES FOR MEN

Obviously there will be some overlap between men and women who may experience arousal and pleasure from similar techniques and styles of self-pleasuring.

Here are a few ideas about ways men can self-pleasure. As with women there are many different ways and each person can find their own styles through experimenting.

Hand techniques

These largely involve causing friction against the frenulum, that part of the penis just under the glans head of the penis. It is highly concentrated in nerve endings which mean it is designed for sensual pleasure (like the clitoris in the woman).

Hand styles vary according to how many fingers are used, how lightly they stimulate, strength of pressure, speed of movement and whether the foreskin is used (if present).

Some men use the whole hand around the penis, sliding or pumping up and down using the friction of the foreskin being moved up and down for extra pleasure. A common way using fingers is to place the thumb and two fingers around the corona (that very sensitive part of the penis just below the penis head) with another finger over the frenulum and rub up and down at whatever speed is the most enjoyable.

Massaging or rubbing the penis head with the palm of your hand or fingers can be very arousing. This can be aided, as can the other styles, by using lubricants such as saliva or oils or creams. You may find if you are circumcised that you need or like to use a lubricant, perhaps something with a slightly astringent effect for a tingling sensation, such as aftershave or hair mousse, but use carefully as irritation or pain may occur.

Beginning Again Alone

Some men like to stimulate their testicles, for example, caressing them, holding them or pulling them away from the body with one hand while pleasuring their penis with the other.

Touching, caressing the anal area and insertion of finger/fingers into the anus can be arousing.

Using the whole body – touching and caressing all over can be very stimulating before centring on more erotic areas.

You can self-pleasure in many positions – standing up, crouching, sitting down, lying on your front or back, kneeling.

Other methods
Water pressure is a pleasurable method, using the pressure from the shower hose or bath taps directly against sensitive areas.

Try friction against other objects or surfaces – for example, lying on your front and rubbing your groin against bedclothes or pillow, either clothed or naked. Use a soft sensuous material, such as a silk scarf or cotton knickers or shirt (for additional stimulation of body smells), against the penis shaft or around glans head.

Sexual toys: some men use a vibrator all over the body as a general turn-on, then use it more directly on the penis, testicles or anus. Again, it may be wrapped in some sensuous material for added effect.

Using a tie or belt tied around the scrotum and penis shaft can also provide erotic stimulation. Some men try cock rings which when put on the penis can increase eroticism.

Try not to be erection- or orgasm-oriented when you self-pleasure. If you are just concerned with producing a hard-as-rock erection then this may intrude into the enjoyment you are giving yourself. It is possible to climax without an erection anyway – the size and strength of your erection is not necessarily the indicator of how turned on you are; just tune in to the pleasurable feelings you are having.

Do not forget the need for imagination and creativity. Fantasy can play as important a role as you wish. You are the creator and *you* are in control and you do not have to tell them to anyone else.

Do not worry if the methods of self-pleasuring you use have not been mentioned in either of these short lists. Your ways are just as valid because they belong to you and give you pleasure. You may like to try other ways for experimentation to see whether you can make self-pleasuring even more diverse and rewarding.

Self-pleasuring is about being you and sharing your sexuality first with yourself. If you can be sensual with yourself this will probably carry over into your relationships with others. But basically it is for you and is an assertion of your own eroticism. Yes, it has its limits – it may not satisfy your desires to touch, love, snuggle up to, be erotic with another person; these may be strong needs which you are hoping to satisfy.

MASTURBATION AND SELF-ESTEEM

It is very hard to give yourself pleasure, sexually or otherwise, if you do not like yourself or your body. Self-pleasuring depends on you feeling positive and relaxed about you. If you do not feel you are worthy of receiving pleasure or can only receive when another person is giving to you then perhaps you need to stop, take stock and start feeling better about yourself (more about this in Chapter 6). It may be that you find it easy to care for yourself in other ways, for example, personal treats, relaxation, interests, asking for support from friends, but do not feel quite right about treating yourself sexually. If so, perhaps you should ask yourself why; try and define the barriers but go ahead anyway.

You might like to try this exercise:

> EXERCISE: *Self-pleasuring II*
> Try and create a similar sensual atmosphere as with the original self-pleasuring experience. Make sure you have time and privacy and warmth.
>
> – Pleasure yourself all over with oil, lotion or powder, as before. Don't rush this – return to areas you find most sensitive and enjoy stimulating them. You may fantasize while you are pleasuring.
> – When you are ready, move to the erotic areas which you find the most pleasing for you. Your sensations will become stronger as the sexual tension mounts – you can quicken up or slow down according to your likes. Use other stimuli such as sexy thoughts, pictures, music, clothing, light, smells to help you focus in on your pleasure. If you want to go on to orgasm then do – tune in and let yourself go.

In this chapter we have been looking at being alone and trying to challenge some of the old myths, assumptions and negative labels with which the status of being on your own is often associated. You can be alone but self-knowing, self-caring and sexual – a nice state in its own right and a good basis to being with a partner should you want to be with one.

6

Beginning Again with a Partner

Turning the theory of safer sex into practice with a partner requires a commitment to the principle of safer sex, a willingness to share your commitment with a partner, the ability to deal calmly and assertively with their responses, and finally and perhaps most important some good, basic communication skills.

If you are not really committed to making a place for safer sex in your life, you are going to be easily dissuaded, so why bother even trying? On the other hand if you are committed, then it will be because you have a solid sense of self-respect and self-worth together with the ability to treat your partners with the same respect with which you yourself would like to be treated.

Self-esteem

Security and self-esteem seem to be most enduring when they come mainly from within yourself rather than being dependent on the goodwill of others. If your sense of self-worth depends on your friends, family, colleagues or partners, you are going to be reluctant to jeopardize this. Consequently you are probably going to do things you do not want, agree to things with which you disagree, and generally keep the lid on some negative feelings. If you do resist the urge to say the things you need to say to people because you fear losing their approval, you are going to be in a very vulnerable situation! If this rings bells for you, it might be worth considering the origins of this low self-esteem.

This might result from experiences in your early childhood and be a general pattern in your life, or else it may be the result of a temporary setback which you have perceived as a failure on your part. If it is the latter, then time will restore your self-esteem and you can use this time to consider how the setback came about, what you might do to avoid it happening again, and what you have learned from the experience.

If your low self-esteem results from experiences in childhood you may need to do more work to resolve the situation. Apart from resorting to professional help from a counsellor, you could begin this work by working out your personal strengths and weaknesses.

How you deal with your partner depends very much on the nature of your relationship. For instance, if you have only just met then this will inevitably be different from dealing with a partner in a long-standing relationship. What seems to matter here is the ability to balance respect (and many other feelings) for your partner, together with respect for yourself. If you are to attempt to deal with partners you will need patience and to be prepared for the possibility of conflict. It is with these things in mind that the communication skills in this chapter are presented.

We do not believe that the problems that face us in

Safer Sex

> EXERCISE: Personal Inventory
>
> You do this by writing two lists: one with all the positives you can think of about yourself, the other with your weaknesses. You need to be as specific as possible if this is going to be of any help to you. So rather than saying for instance, 'I'm shy', you could identify the kinds of situations that make you more likely to feel uncomfortable and behave in a shy manner. You will then be more able to identify some goals for yourself.
>
> Then take the negatives you have identified and turn them from negatives into goals you want to achieve. For instance your negatives might include 'I'm uncomfortable with strangers' or 'I don't feel confident expressing my point of view', so you would change these to: 'I want to be more comfortable with strangers' or 'I want to feel confident about expressing my point of view'.
>
> Once you've identified your goals, you give them priority according to the degree of difficulty you anticipate in achieving them. So you begin with one that will be relatively easy to change. It is important that you do not sabotage yourself by setting your sights impossibly high. That will only lead to a sense of failure, confirming your poor self-image. Then take your goal and break it down into small manageable steps, addressing these one by one and assessing how you are doing as you go. If you cannot manage the step you have set yourself, it was the *step* that was to blame, not *you*, so simply break it down further until you can achieve it.

our sexual lives are overcome simply by reading a book about it. We can only help you to draw the map – you are the one making the journey.

Communicating effectively

Effective communication is a question of saying what you mean and meaning what you say. In other words, it means sending the message you intend to send and receiving the message that is sent.

Over the years we have all evolved a number of ways of communicating, some learned from our parents, others picked up along the way. The problem for many of us is that we did not have good role models from whom we could learn communication skills. Instead we learned a variety of ways of getting what we wanted. We learned to manipulate rather than to communicate, by being dishonest, not declaring feelings, lying, putting ourselves or other people down, being silent, being too 'nice', using jargon or intellectualizing – all ways of avoiding clear communication.

Part of the difficulty with these styles of communicating is that they prevent rather than bring about intimacy. Intimacy is risky, it means not only enjoying the good things together but being able to share the difficult things also. Doing this is easier if we can learn more effective ways of communicating together which will bring us closer instead of driving a wedge between us and the people we are trying to get close to.

Essentially this means being able to distinguish thoughts from feelings, and expressing each appropriately, and making sure that both verbal and non-verbal messages are the same, rather than conflicting with each other. When you can do this, you will be more able to express your feelings, needs and wishes clearly and directly, without relying on your partner's extrasensory perception! You will also be more able and confident about saying 'yes' and 'no', and about dealing with conflict creatively rather than aggressively or defensively.

Safer Sex

GROUND RULES FOR EFFECTIVE COMMUNICATION

To begin developing these skills you will need some basic groundrules.

1. Effective communication is based on mutual respect, trust and above all the ability and willingness to listen.
2. If we are responsible for expressing our own thoughts and feelings, then we can show that we are doing this by using what is called 'I' language. An example of this would be to say 'I am feeling angry' rather than 'you're making me angry' or 'I am too busy' instead of 'you're not giving me enough time'.
3. *You* are responsible for expressing your needs and wishes.
4. You are *not* responsible for *what* you are feeling. We all have feelings all of the time. We cannot stop ourselves feeling, but we can take responsibility for what we do with that feeling.

FEELINGS

The first thing we need to do is to sort out the difference between our thoughts and our feelings. Thoughts are what go on in our head. Feelings are more difficult to describe, but people often talk about feelings as coming from their gut (gut reaction). Feelings may not be easy to have sometimes, but they are relatively simple to express as they can usually be expressed in one word, for example 'I feel sad', 'I feel happy' or 'I feel angry'. When you find yourself saying things like: 'I feel I'm going to go mad' you're not actually expressing the feeling, but the thought that accompanies it.

Sex is simply one aspect of our lives and relationships, and will inevitably be influenced by whatever else is going on in our lives and relationships. So if we have had a lousy day, or a row with a lover, it would be, for

Beginning Again with a Partner

most of us, very unrealistic to expect to be able immediately to put this to one side and make love together in perfect harmony! Whatever is left unresolved in the rest of our lives and relationships is likely to follow us into our sexual relationships.

It might seem threatening to begin looking at this aspect of your life and relationships, but we are inevitably communicating anyway, and this section is designed to help you to assess whether you might do this more effectively.

All of us have feelings all the time. Much as we might like to ignore or hide them at times, they are important and very real. They influence all our lives and we need to develop a way of dealing with them. We might choose to ignore them, but if we do this they are going to make their presence known anyway, often out of our control (the 'last straw' syndrome when something trivial acts as the trigger for the release of an accumulated backlog of anger).

Alternatively, we might decide to abdicate our responsibility for them and instead dump them on our partners, for instance by saying things like 'you're making me feel . . .' The problem with this is threefold. First, they are not making you feel anything; the feelings are within you, nobody put them there. Second, if they are having to deal in this way with your feelings, they are not going to get time to deal with their own, and you may then get these dumped back onto you. Third, they are likely to feel angry and resentful (in addition to what they were feeling) and this is hardly likely to help them either respect or want to get close to you.

So what can you do? You can decide that your feelings are your responsibility, and that you are in charge of their expression. You could begin by allowing yourself to simply have and experience feelings, allowing them to occur without censorship. This is often more of an issue for men who are brought up to believe that feelings are a sign of weakness and failure, and that talking about them is a measure of their inadequacy. Sensitivity to both our own and our partners' feelings can never be a bad thing. If we will not get in touch with our own feelings, we are closing ourselves off from a fundamental part of our existence. We are also closing ourselves off from those around us. Nobody wants to get close to a robot!

Having allowed ourselves to get in touch with our feelings, we then have to decide what we are going to do with them. We talked earlier about ignoring them, or else dumping them onto others and suggested some potential consequences of this. Another thing we can do is to turn them in our ourselves. For example, when we are angry with someone we can decide not to let them know and instead take the anger out on ourselves. This is often an issue for women who are led to believe that they should not have negative feelings because these are at odds with their role as 'carers' and 'nurturers'. They then turn those negative feelings in on themselves and depression may be the result. The other difficulty with this is that apart from the fact that they hinder rather than help closeness, they do not effectively resolve conflict or bad feeling and lead instead to an accumulation of feelings which will eventually need to be sorted out.

So what you do is begin by recognizing and acknowledging how you feel, simply and clearly, using the 'I' language discussed above. So if you were feeling angry you might say 'I'm feeling angry' which is much clearer than either 'you're making me feel angry' or 'I feel that you/he/she/they shouldn't have done ...' (whatever it was that led to you becoming angry). Remember to avoid the word 'that' as in 'I feel that ...' using this you

Beginning Again with a Partner

are expressing a thought and not a feeling.

The next step is for you to have your feeling recognized and acknowledged by your partner. Feelings are not rational and however 'silly' they may seem, they are all too real and important to us when we are feeling them. Being told we are being 'stupid' or 'childish' is only going to make us feel worse. What we need to hear is that someone accepts how we feel. So your partner might say 'I'm sorry you feel like that'. They then have a chance to express how they feel. When you have acknowledged, expressed and accepted how each other feels, with the feelings out in the open you are going to be in a better position to deal with the situation. The next step is to discuss your thoughts and see if you can come to some acceptable negotiation or conclusion.

BODY LANGUAGE

Very often communication becomes unclear because we send people mixed messages. Not only is it important that we say what we mean and mean what we say, but we should also *look* as if we mean it. For instance, saying that you are angry with someone when you are smiling disguises your anger and might leave them feeling bewildered as to what you actually mean. Another example would be talking about closeness but with your arms folded around yourself and your legs crossed, which gives altogether a different message.

ASSERTION SKILLS

An important ingredient of communication skills is the ability to be assertive. This is not the same as being aggressive. It means your ability to be responsible for yourself, to allow others to be responsible for themselves, and to treat yourself and those around you with respect. This means that you allow yourself to say what you think, want and need, to make mistakes, to change your mind, to say 'yes' and 'no', and face up to conflict instead of avoiding it.

You can see that one of the key differences between assertion and aggression is that aggression is based on a lack of respect for others. Assertive behaviour does not result in 'loss of face' for anyone, and so is more likely to lead to an acceptable outcome. When people get aggressive it becomes a question of 'winning' and 'losing'. Assertion allows both people to be in a 'win' position. When people realize that there is no competition they are less likely to respond competitively. Therefore the issue does not get lost in the 'battle'.

So how do you go about being more assertive? If you are using the communication skills outlined above you are halfway there already. Using 'I' language, rather than saying 'it' 'you' or 'we', is an open declaration that you are taking responsibility for what you are saying, rather than dumping this onto others.

You might also have to change some of the words you use. For instance if you have got into the habit of saying '*can't*' when you really mean '*won't*' you are sending an ambiguous message. So instead of saying 'I can't see you tonight' say 'I won't see you tonight'. Become aware of whether when you say '*should*' what you really mean to say is '*choose to*' or '*could*'. When you say 'should' you are denying your own responsibility and autonomy. Similarly when you say 'need' do you really *mean* 'need' or 'would like' or 'want': when you say 'I *need* something to drink' you might be meaning 'I *want* something to drink'. If so, say so.

Demonstrating your responsibility for yourself is also possible by using words that imply you 'do' or 'are' things, rather than that things simply happen *to* you. For instance, I might say that my mother always calls me to tell me her problems, when what I really mean is that I *allow* her to ring me and tell me all her problems.

Another important point in assertion is about asking questions as a hidden way of stating an opinion. So I might say 'don't you think that he's really boring', when what I would say if I were assertive would be either 'I think he's boring' (if I want to state an opinion), or 'what do you think of him' (if I genuinely want to find out your opinion of him).

PUTTING IT INTO PRACTICE

You may well be reading this and thinking, 'this is all very well but how the hell am I going to put this into practice in my relationship?'

Again, there are some guidelines you can follow. To begin with pick your moment carefully. It is probably not a wise idea to decide when you are with a group of friends that now is the time to sort out your sexual relationship. You may need to make a request to set aside some time to talk. You might decide to tackle some less threatening aspects of your relationships first before approaching the sexual arena. There is a good reason for this. Many people invest a considerable amount of their self-esteem in their sexuality and are therefore quick to feel attacked, threatened or undermined, and interpret any discussion of sexual matters as a personal slight.

You may be prepared to say things that are perhaps difficult to say, but are you ready to *hear* things that may be difficult to hear without becoming defensive or argumentative? If so, you can agree with your partner that it probably will not be very easy to communicate in this way to begin with, but if you persevere you will have gone a long way towards making your relationship stronger. Help each other out if you get stuck. You will probably not get it right immediately, but if you can assist each other you are more likely to succeed.

Of course there is always the possibility that when you begin looking a little more closely at your relationship you find yourselves opening a can of worms – here perhaps a willing third party may help. Marriage guidance counsellors and therapists see people who are single, coupled, married or not. They do not have any vested interest in keeping your relationship together. If you find that the best solution is for you to separate, painful as this may be, professional help might enable you to do this with dignity instead of an endless stream of recriminations.

Let us assume that you are beginning to get the hang of it by now. The first period of trying out this new style of communication may be difficult because you may have to deal with a backlog of unexpressed resentments and other negative feelings. You can take comfort from the fact that in future you are going to be able to deal with issues as and when they occur, and so will not be afraid of a hangover of bad feeling. You can learn to trust that each of you will say whatever you need to say *when* you need to say it.

It is also important that you do not interpret the resolution of conflict as meaning that you have to compromise every single time. For instance, one of you might want some gentle massage and the other some more aggressive sexual play. If you compromise with some aggressive sexual massage, you may find neither of you gets what you want! Why not agree on time for each? This will mean that both of you are in a 'win' position. If you are making compromises all the time, rather than trying to make sure that each of you gets what you want, you are going to find yourselves getting only part of what you want and possibly feeling resentful into the bargain!

As you can see assertion and communication are skills which take time and practice to learn. You may want to join a group to get some support as you acquire these skills (details in Appendix 1). Once you are confident that you can deal with your feelings, and that conflict is being addressed in your relationship whenever it occurs, you may now be ready to turn your attention to the sexual side of your relationship.

Finding a sexual language

Sexual relationships have seldom been easy to negotiate in our society because of the difficulties we have with the whole subject. We still have not found a language for talking about sex that is not too medical for some people or offensive to others. Maybe this is the whole problem – maybe there cannot ever be *one* sexual language, but rather a variety from which we can choose the one with which we feel most comfortable.

The language we use reveals a lot about how we feel. Sexuality has a most elaborate range of language relating to it: from medical and scientific terminology, to the beauty of literature to the earthiness of colloquiallism. Some of the words used for the male and female genitals, masturbation, oral sex and sexual intercourse are given below. Consider as you read them the images they convey for you.

Safer Sex

MALE GENITALS
Penis, scrotum, testicles, cock, prick, tool, family jewels, balls, gones, nuts, dick, dong, joystick, meat, organ, pecker, poker, rod, privates, sword, magic wand, john thomas, dipstick, lady's delight, knob, prong, sausage, pipe, phallus, sack, dingus, quim wedge, baby-maker, weapon, one-eyed trouser snake, club, joint, skin flute, willy, pistol, rocket, hot dog, hampton wick, percy, bishop, canary, hammer, winkle, relic, old man, member, orchids, marbles, bollocks, knackers, bags, basket, groceries, lunch, goolies, cobblers, pills, jumbucks.

FEMALE GENITALS
Cunt, fanny, beaver, minge, honeypot, slit, crack, hole, pussy, twat, mousetrap, jelly roll, bearded clam, snatch, quim, cooch, gash, muff, bearded lady, manhole, toolbox, coozy, doughnut, love hole, furburger, vagina, pudenda, vulva, goalie, button, clit.

BREASTS
Tits, paps, bazookas, funbags, boobs, bosom, bust, bristols, cans, knockers, chest, melons, grapefruits, headlights.

MASTURBATION
Wank, jerk off, play pocket billiards, toss off, beat the meat, pound the pud, beat the bishop, wack off, have one off on the wrist, milk, punish percy in the palm, finger job, hand job, hand jive, hand shandy, J arthur rank, wrist job, dollop the weaner, pull the pudding, playing chopsticks, have a date with a handkerchief, the housewife's hour.

Beginning Again with a Partner

ORAL SEX

Drop on it, blow job, give head, get a facial, inhale the oyster, polish the knob, head job, take it in the mouth, cock-sucking, deep throat, knob job, plating, cunt-sucking/munching, frenching, going down, pussy nibbling, cake eater, cat lapper, muff diving, tonguing.

INTERCOURSE

Have sex, sleep with, fuck, hump, shag, screw, roll in the hay, fool around, get it on, get into someone's pants, lay, give one to, bunk up, ball, score, have the banana peeled, dip the wick, get the leg over, shaft, make, poke, service, bang, pump, have it off, have it away, have a bit of the other.

These terms give some idea of the range of very vivid language available to describe sex. What do you mainly notice about these words? Why do so many of them relate to men? Are there differences between the words for male and female genitals? If so, what are they?

If you are struggling to find a sexual language to use with your partner you might agree to both read this list (adding any words of your own) and (separately) underline those you find acceptable, then swap lists. It is important to be direct with each other about those words you find offensive or unacceptable, since hearing these words used either when you are talking about or having sex is going to be a distraction for you. If you find it very difficult to even say any of these words, you might like to read the lists out alone, noting how, and to which words you react most/least favourably. This will give you the beginning of your own sexual vocabulary. Remember that if you cannot find *any* of these words acceptable, you can always, alone or with a partner, invent your own words for your private use.

Sexual communication

When it comes to sexual communication there are several things to consider: making sexual statements, making requests, dealing with conflict and negotiation. Let us look at each of these in turn.

A survey carried out by *Woman* magazine a few years ago revealed some interesting details of the sexual lives of their respondents. Among them were the facts that: over fifty per cent of their unmarried respondents said they found it difficult to talk freely to their partners about sex; only a third of the wives could talk openly to their husbands about sex, while another third avoided making sexual requests; additionally more than a third regularly agreed to practices that they did not enjoy and which made them feel uneasy. According to another more recent survey carried out by *She* magazine, more than one-fifth of their respondents have sex with their partners in total silence.

Apart from the fact that an inability to talk about sex is linked (unsurprisingly) to sexual problems, if we are relying on our partner's extrasensory perception to know how to please us sexually this may be easier, but more often than not we are going to be disappointed! So if we are reluctant to talk about sex we are not very likely to get what we want, and are therefore potentially depriving ourselves of pleasure. Also many people like to hear what pleases their partner, so you are not only depriving yourself you may also be depriving your partner. Many people find noisy sex a turn-on. You might now like to think about what happens when you have sex with your partner. Are there things you would like to say but feel inhibited about?

An important aspect of sexual communication is being able to ask for what we want. Having developed and applied the communication skills above we may now be better placed to ask for what we want, because we will be able to recognize that this is our responsibility and it seems the most likely way of getting what we want. For instance applying the guidelines above, we might be saying things like 'I'd like you to take off my clothes' instead of 'you never take off my clothes'.

Dealing with conflict becomes a little less threatening when we make use of the guidelines on assertion and communication above. In addition to those skills here are some other hints to consider. You are probably going to have more chance of resolving a situation if you are positive rather than negative (for example 'I'd love it if you ...', instead of 'you never ...'). Also you are more likely to be successful if you join together for instance, 'what are *we* going to do about this?' rather than 'well, what are *you* going to do then?' Make sure you acknowledge what the other person is saying. If you are not sure what they mean, do not make assumptions, ask them to clarify. Be creative together in looking at possible solutions. You could agree to look at *all* the possible outcomes, however undesirable or unrealistic, so that you can then choose those that are acceptable, realistic and desirable, and that take into account *both* your needs.

If you find yourself in a sexual situation when you want to say 'no' to someone what do you do? Do you say 'yes' and go along resentfully? Or say 'no' but behave in a way (for example, smiling, or winking) that might indicate you are unsure or open to persuasion?

Do you:

– use the 'I've got a headache/I'm too tired' routine
– get mad and shout 'fuck off' aggressively
– look them in the eye and say 'no', clearly and non-apologetically

You may be thinking 'that's fine with a stranger or someone you've just met, but it's not so easy with my regular partner: they're going to feel rejected'. Well they might feel rejected. It may be very difficult for you to accept that you are not responsible for how they feel; you did not put those feelings there. Of course if you care about them you are going to be concerned. You cannot take away their feelings, but what you can do is listen and accept what they say without judging them. If you can do this you are treating them with respect, however difficult it may be for each of you. If on the other hand you withdraw your request or agree to theirs the minute they become upset, you're 'rescuing' them from their difficult feelings. If you do this, in effect what you are doing is depriving them of a chance to deal with the issue. You are also denying the validity of your own needs, and in the process, putting them in a powerful position over you.

They might be pleased to hear you being assertive. They might be angry because they are not getting their own way as they always have. Difficult as that may be they are going to have to get used to it. They will have to learn to treat you with the respect you are demonstrating you have for yourself. If you say 'yes' when you mean 'no' not only are you giving a mixed message, you are showing your lack of respect for yourself.

Negotiating safer sex

Now let us look at how we might apply this in relation to safer sex within two contexts: a new relationship, and an ongoing one.

WITH A NEW PARTNER

If you are going to raise the issue with a new partner you should be prepared for a variety of reactions. They may be relieved it was you who mentioned it first and eagerly go along with any suggestions you have. Alternatively they may interpret your concern as implying that there is something wrong either with you or with them. They may think you are being unnecessarily cautious.

If you are in a situation with someone when it seems likely that sex will occur, then it is wise to mention safer sex before anything sexual begins, so that you can make a dignified retreat if necessary. It is not a wise idea to leave it till the last minute when you have got your clothes off before suggesting a condom is used! It is wise to have a clear head when you are talking about it. Drugs and alcohol in this instance may leave you with more than a hangover. Where do you begin?

You need to have sorted out for yourself in advance what your thoughts and feelings are on the issue, so that you can be prepared for any conflict or discussion that arises.

It may be easier to be assertive with someone you do not know very well. What have you got to lose if sex does not happen? Only the fantasy of what it might have been like. However, it can also be more difficult talking about safer sex with someone you do not know very well. You might worry about how mentioning safer sex makes you appear to them. For instance, you might think carrying condoms around with you makes you look as if you are always on the lookout for a quick screw. We might worry about rejection or the possibility of an argument.

If you have decided for yourself that safer sex is what you want, and you have practised being assertive in other aspects of your life, you are probably going to be more successful. Here is a demonstration of how you can use the principle of assertion to help you. You might like to rehearse this in your head substituting the kind of words you would use in this situation.

- I'd really like to have sex with you. I have a rule for myself that if I fuck I always use a condom.

instead of:

- We've got to use a condom because I don't know what you might pass on to me.

Let us say the partner responds by saying:

- Look, there's nothing wrong with me, all this stuff about safer sex is only for people who *really* sleep around.

a suitable response could be:

- I don't know what *really* sleeping around means. As I said, I'd like to have sex with you, and I want us to use a condom.

the partner might then get a little more aggressive:

- Are you saying I might give you something, is that what you mean?

response:

- No I'm not saying that you might 'give me something'. I'd like to have sex with you but I have a rule for *myself* about condoms, do you appreciate what I am saying?

As you can see from this example the assertive partner states a wish/thought/feeling, listens to the other's reply, responds accordingly, but repeats as often as necessary his/her initial wish/thought/feeling, checking out that the other person has understood. You can decide for yourself how a scenario like this might end if

Beginning Again with a Partner

you were one of the partners. Imagine yourself in both roles and think about how you might respond. Would you give in, become aggressive or agree? You might like to take this further, by working out for yourself some examples of situations relating to safer sex that you are likely to come across, and then consider how you might handle them assertively.

How long you go on dealing with objections or resistance will depend on you: how committed you are to the idea of safer sex, how much you like the other person, how much patience you have, and possibly how creative you both are in coming up with some interesting solutions to your dilemma!

With partners who complain that safer sex is boring you might find yourself in the position of having to use your powers of persuasion, and offering some imaginative challenges to their assumptions about safer sex. For instance you might say 'Let's see if I can get a condom on to you without using my hands'.

Again, if you are to get anywhere, it is important that it should be a 'win-win' situation. So if you cannot agree about using condoms for instance, you might each offer some safer sexual alternatives you would really enjoy and see if you can agree on those!

This is not to say that you must be successful every time. The important thing is to be able to learn from the times when things do not go according to plan, and work out how you might approach it differently the next time.

IN AN ONGOING RELATIONSHIP

With partners where you have established a relationship the issue may be easier, or possibly more difficult: easier because you know each other, trust each other and treat each other respectfully enough to take seriously anything you both want to discuss; more difficult because talking about relationships is seldom easy, particularly when talking about sex, and even more so when you're talking about previous sexual experiences, activities, partners, and the possibility of making changes.

You may be wondering what, if anything, safer sex has to do with you: 'If you're in a monogamous relationship you don't have to worry about HIV'. A number of things must be taken into account here. For one thing monogamous relationships do end. Some people then begin another monogamous relationship, what is called 'serial monogamy'. The difficulty is that even monogamy is no absolute guarantee against infection. Unless we know *for certain* that neither partner has or could have HIV (or any other infection for that matter) and trust each other not to become infected through the course of a relationship, safer sex is certainly an issue to consider. According to the well-publicized sex research of the last decade *The Hite Report* (see Appendix 3) nearly three-quarters of the married men respondents reported having had sex with someone other than their wife. The other surveys we mentioned earlier similarly reveal that approximately four out of ten unmarried women had had sex with a married man, and four out of ten of the married women had had sex with someone other than their husband.

This is not intended to sow seeds of doubt in anyone's mind but simply to remind us that not everyone finds it possible to live up to the expectation of monogamy and that the social unacceptability of 'infidelity' or 'sexually open relationships' can make it difficult to admit to sex outside an ongoing relationship. If we have these doubts even after discussing the issue with partners, safer sex is practical protection available to us all.

Beginning Again with a Partner

If you are going to discuss safer sex with your partner choose a time when you will be free from interruptions and when you are both reasonably calm. Trying to discuss safer sex in bed before you go to sleep after a hard day is probably not a wise idea. Similarly, mentioning it as you go on the bus to a friend's house might not be very productive! You will both need time, patience and a commitment to listen.

Create an atmosphere where you are going to be able to talk in a relaxed unhurried fashion. Then using the guidelines above you might begin by saying 'I'd like to talk with you about safer sex'. It is important not to allow yourself to be distracted by jokes or putdowns. It is also important that you allow your partner sufficient time to take in what you are saying, think about it, express how he/she feels, ask questions and respond.

You may find that if you are good at communicating with each other that it becomes a matter of 'forget the "whether", let's talk about *what* and *when!*' If you are able to present your case positively and creatively you are going to be more successful than if you are full of doom and gloom and waving AIDS leaflets.

You must also consider the possibility that no amount of persuasion, assertion, and pleading on your part will get your partner to consider the issue. If this is the case it might reflect an inability or refusal on their part to respect your wishes and needs. Only you can decide for yourself if you want to remain in a relationship like this.

It is often difficult to make changes. The risk of upsetting or even losing partners we care about is threatening to most of us. The risk of not saying what we want or need to say for fear of losing them, may force us to pay a higher price – higher perhaps than we might care to imagine.

7

Safer Sexual Intercourse?

Sexual intercourse is, of course, simply one way of being sexual together. However, because it is a very important activity for many people, and because it is also a very effective way of transmitting infections, this chapter is concerned with helping you to identify for yourself what role, if any, sexual intercourse should have in your sexual life, and how you might make it safer for yourself. You should read this chapter and Chapter 8 together because these two chapters deal specifically with the practicalities of safer sex.

Although in the next chapter we shall look a little more closely at what the phrase 'sexual intercourse' might mean, in this section we shall assume that it refers to penetrative sex involving the penis inserted into the vagina or anus.

It is important to stress that the decision whether, or how, to have intercourse is one that only you can make for yourself. It is often difficult, as we hope we have shown throughout this book, to be rational about sex. Now, more than ever, we need to be responsible for

Safer Sexual Intercourse?

ourselves, and this means paying attention to both our thoughts and our feelings. This is what the rest of this chapter is about.

Why do you want to have intercourse?

Let us think for a moment about some of the reasons people might offer for having or wanting sexual intercourse.

- They enjoy it
- They think it is the most natural way to have sex
- They want to be physically close
- They want to have a child
- They think intercourse reinforces their definitions of themselves as masculine and feminine
- They enjoy the feeling of power intercourse gives them
- They enjoy the sensations of the penis in the vagina/ anus
- They are lonely
- They want sexual pleasure
- They want to have an orgasm
- They do not want to have to think about other ways of being sexual together
- They want to be 'intimate'
- They are randy
- They have never thought that sex might mean anything else

Of course the list is endless, it has to be because we are all so different. Perhaps you might like to make up your own list based on the reasons why you have had or wanted intercourse. The point is that many of the reasons listed here might lead to other sensual or sexual activities if we accepted that these are acceptable alternatives. For instance being randy or wanting to come or be intimate or close, might, if we allowed it, lead to other things happening between us and our partners. For example, we might like to hug each other when we want closeness, or to be masturbated when we want to come or to have sex in some of the ways described in the next chapter.

Women often find that by itself intercourse provides insufficient stimulation for them to have an orgasm. In fact nearly two-thirds of women are unable to have an orgasm from the stimulation produced by intercourse alone. The fact that the clitoris is outside and a little away from the vagina means that most women have to have additional clitoral stimulation to have an orgasm during intercourse.

Men also report some drawbacks to intercourse. In our culture intercourse is practically the only time men allow themselves to get physically close to women. However it might be good for both women and men if intercourse happens because it is a definite choice instead of a necessity or expectation whenever they feel sexual.

Some men find that they feel pressurized by intercourse: to have an erection, to be able to delay ejaculation, and simultaneously to provide their partner with extra stimulation. Little wonder then that many men and women report their strongest orgasms when they masturbate, since they can then give themselves the kind of stimulation they like, and are relatively free from the anxiety of having to 'perform' for anyone else.

Our culture sees sex as 'guilty till proven innocent', therefore we need to justify it, and what better justification than having children? This might help explain the illegality of anal intercourse between heterosexuals since

Safer Sexual Intercourse?

by its nature it is non-reproductive sex. It seems that the fact that most acts of intercourse do not result in pregnancy is conveniently ignored. This whole question of how we became so hooked on intercourse as the only 'real' kind of sex could take up a whole book of its own.

However, for our purposes, if we relegate any other kind of sexual activity apart from penis in vagina to 'just foreplay' or 'not real sex' we are saying that these activities are not enjoyable and valuable in their own right.

Also in relegating to the ranks of 'preliminaries' or 'foreplay' any sexual activity that does not consist of penetration, we have made a rod for our own backs, since it is essentially *these* activities that form the basis of safer sex. Apart from the risk of infection, the emphasis on penetrative sex robs many people of the experience of finding other ways of being sexual together. We might like to consider how important intercourse is for us as individuals, and the possibility that we might have tended to ignore the erotic potential of 'non-penetrative' sex.

EXERCISE: *Sexual Inventory*

Think back over your sexual life, and see if there was ever a time that you agreed to have intercourse when you did not really want it. Try to picture the scene quite clearly and just think about what happened for a few minutes. Did you have any idea of what you wanted to do sexually with this person? Did you let your partner know? Did they put you down/ignore you/persuade you? What was it that allowed you to go ahead with intercourse you did not want? Was it the fear of being laughed at/thought weird or kinky/of not being 'normal'/or the wish to please your partner? Finally, if this situation occurred again would you approach it differently this time, and if so how?

The point of the exercise above is not to leave you feeling guilty, but rather to help you identify whether or not you need to become clearer about what role intercourse has in your sexual life. As we have said already intercourse has seldom, if ever, been entirely risk-free. HIV has become one more, albeit very serious consideration to weigh up when you're deciding what role if any intercourse has in your sexual life.

If you have already decided that intercourse is not always going to be part of your sexual repertoire, then read Chapter 8 which concerns itself with other examples of safer sex for you to think about.

But if you *are* having, or are intending to have intercourse, please read on because the next section deals with the subject of condoms, which can help to make intercourse safer. But do read Chapter 8 as well because it might help you to find a way of sorting out your sexual and sensual preferences and priorities and of seeing intercourse as simply one of a range of sexual alternatives.

Condoms

Having decided that intercourse is going to be a part of your sexual life, from the point of view of safety you need to think about protecting yourself and your partners with a condom.

The role of condoms in preventing sexually transmitted diseases was known to our ancestors many centuries ago who used them primarily for this purpose. The issue of condoms to soldiers during the Second World War led to a huge reduction in the rate of sexual infections and pregnancies and highlighted the dramatic preventive possibilities of the condom.

Safer Sexual Intercourse?

The introduction of more convenient methods of contraception together with the availability of relatively effective treatments for sexually transmitted diseases resulted in the declining popularity of the condom.

One of the results of this is that many men were able to hand over responsibility for birth control to women, and women were able to assume responsibility for their own contraception. Many people became used to the idea of sex without 'barriers'. In turn this reinforced notions of sex as being 'spontaneous' uninterrupted by the nuisance of fiddling about looking for and putting on a condom. Getting used to condoms again means that we need to discover ways of including them as just another part of sex; in other words we need to find ways of making condoms erotic.

The media hype about herpes earlier this decade, together with the increasing incidence of strains of gonorrhoea resistant to penicillin, cervical cancer and of course HIV has led to a high level of interest in the preventive possibilities of the humble condom. Indeed for many safer sex campaigns, condoms *are* safer sex. However, there is a bit more to it than that. Condoms do not make sex *safe*, just less risky. How effective they are depends on two factors: the reliability of the condom and the reliability of you, the users.

A condom acts as a barrier. This very fine barrier is sufficient to preserve sensation while protecting partners from the potentially undesirable consequences of infection or pregnancy. And maybe the most important question is about infection *or* pregnancy.

It is really important to be clear about *why* you might be introducing condoms into your safer sex life. People often confuse the contraceptive qualities of a condom with the hygienic ones, but it is more complicated than that.

Safer Sex

If you have used condoms in the past because you wanted to avoid pregnancy you will have thought through the options and presumably chosen the condom because it is the method that suits you best. All the time more and more people are beginning to think about barrier methods of contraception as a viable option as the condom becomes more popular.

The high profile of the now fashionable condom has been in the context of the public health campaign designed to raise awareness about AIDS. If you are one of the many people using condoms as a protection against infection, then it is worthwhile to think about this as a separate issue from protection against pregnancy. For example, imagine that you are using your condom for protection against both infection and pregnancy. The condom breaks – you now have the worry of *both* infection and pregnancy. So if you are using condoms for both purposes you would be advised to consider using another method for contraception (if, of course, you want to avoid a pregnancy).

The confusion between the dual role of condoms is highlighted by those who think that they are 'doing their bit' against infection by using a 'cap', the 'pill', or some other method of contraception.

*It is important to be clear about
why you are using
what you are using*

CHOOSING A CONDOM

Having made your decision to use condoms the first step is of course getting them. But where do you begin? If you prefer you can get them free from family planning clinics. Also some STD clinics are now issuing condoms to clients who request them. But you might not have

Safer Sexual Intercourse?

much choice about how many you get or what kind you are given.

Finding the condom that suits you is a process of trial and error so you might like to try a selection and see which you like best. You can get them from chemists, some large supermarket chains, barbers, slot machines in pubs and clubs, mail order from ads in the personal columns of magazines and newspapers, and of course from sex shops. As we write this moves are afoot to try to make condoms as easily obtainable as newspapers.

The first shop in the world specializing in condoms opened in 1987 in Amsterdam with the aim of offering a relaxing environment for both women and men to see, and select from, the wide range of condoms available on the market.

The most common condoms are those made of latex, but it is also possible to buy condoms made from natural membrane. However, these are expensive and cannot be tested. They are generally considered to be less effective than latex condoms and therefore not of much use as part of safer sex.

How do you begin selecting which ones you might like to try? The variety is considerable. They are available in different thicknesses, shapes, sizes, colours, with or without teats, textured surfaces, flavours, perfumes, with or without lubricant, and with or without an ingredient to delay ejaculation! One company also make a condom specifically for those who have allergic reactions.

It's really a question of finding what suits you best in terms of satisfaction, fit, appearance, and of course effectiveness (and possibly taste, depending on what you are going to do with it!).

Obviously the thinner the condom the less interference there will be with sensitivity. However, this has to be weighed against the likely wear and tear on the condom during sexual activity. Almost all condoms measure somewhere between 0.03mm and 0.09mm. Contrary to what you might think, condoms are *not* all the same size. Brand names can be a good indication as to which men they cater for in terms of penis size. This is a chance to swallow pride and get what is likely to suit you most, instead of clinging to silly stereotypes like 'the bigger the better'. Colours vary from coral to black and most conceivable shades in between.

It is now possible for those who want them to get condoms without teats. Some people feel that the teatless condom is possibly less likely to break and more attractive in appearance. The names of some condoms imply that they provide additional stimulation for the partner at the receiving end of the condom-clad penis. Some people report that they do obtain extra stimulation from these, but others say they are more likely to massage the ego of the condom user!

For oral sex, the taste of the condom is obviously important. Unless you happen to be a rubber enthusiast the taste and smell of rubber is not very popular: hence the introduction of condoms with different tastes and perfumes. If you are prone to allergies be careful as you may react to having a condom in your mouth.

Lubricated or non-lubricated condoms is another option for the consumer to consider. Again this is a matter for individual consideration. In any case remember that the receiving partner may also need some additional lubrication and this should always be water-based such as KY jelly, rather than oil-based like Vaseline, as this can cause the rubber to perish.

From the point of view of effectiveness several new condoms have appeared on the market recently, including those containing spermicide; those which come with an applicator to prevent accidents putting it on; and those which have an adhesive strip to prevent the condom leaking or (if you will pardon the pun) coming off before desired.

Some condoms are appearing specifically designed to use during anal sex. Whichever condom you use it is important to use plenty of lubrication and to top this up regularly. It is also important to seek advice from one of the agencies listed in Appendix 1 if you are not sure about which condom to buy.

One interesting side-effect of the re-emergence of the condom might be its effect on men who ejaculate prematurely. Some condoms are available which contain a small amount of anaesthetic, allowing the user to delay ejaculation (though hopefully not indefinitely!).

SPERMICIDES

Some spermicides, for example those containing nonoxinol 9, can be used to complement a condom because of their likely effect on HIV. The effect of this chemical on the rectal mucosa is not yet clear, and there is no straightforward advice as to whether or not you should use this during anal sex. Some argue that because we do not know what the effects are we should not use it. However, others argue that the risk of transmission of HIV seriously outweighs any possible danger to the rectum.

STANDARDS OF CONDOMS

In 1964 the United Kingdom introduced a British Standard (BS3704) for condoms and the quality of merchandise improved significantly. This standard was updated in 1979 and is again under revision. Condoms that carry the British Standard Kitemark symbol conform to this standard and their production lines are continuously monitored by the British Standards Institution.

However we cannot assume that those condoms which do not carry the Kitemark to be inferior. Imported condoms may well have passed rigorous testing in their country of origin, but the manufacturers may have been reluctant to pay for BSI inspection. You may also see 'BSI approved' on packaging which means that this brand has passed the strict tests laid down by the BSI even though kitemark status may not have been sought. You should also check that any condom you decide to use has an *expiry date* on the packet.

YOU AND YOUR CONDOM

Having got some samples the next step is to try them out. For men who have never used condoms before, or who have forgotten what it is like to use them, it is worth practising with them alone when you masturbate, getting used to both putting them on, and the different sensation. Try different brands to see which you like best in terms of sensation, fit, and appearance. Exact fit is not essential (as long as it is not likely come off!). Those that are tight around the base can act like a 'cock-ring', a device used by some men to maintain or boost their erection.

Begin by opening the packet taking care not to tear the condom with fingernails or jewellery. Holding the teat between thumb and forefinger press out any air before unrolling the condom along the entire length of the erect penis. Uncircumcised men should pull back their foreskin (if they need to) before the condom goes on. When you are used to condoms and ready to involve your partner, make an agreement that this is going to be fun!

Safer Sexual Intercourse?

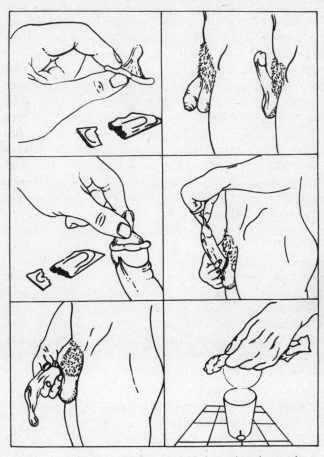

1. Open the packet carefully to avoid damaging the condom.
2. Put the condom on after the penis has become hard.
3. Hold the closed end between the thumb and forefinger to expel the air. 4. Hold the condom over the tip of the penis and unroll it down to the base. 5. After ejaculation withdraw the penis before it becomes soft. Hold the condom firmly around the base of the penis. 6. Slide the condom off and wrap it in a tissue before disposal.

Make sure you have a supply close at hand so you do not have to leap up to go and find one. It might also help to have some soft lighting in the room, because fumbling around in the dark is not only a nuisance but you might mishandle the condom. Play with different colours and textures and take turns practising putting them on and taking them off. It can add sensation to squeeze a drop of KY jelly into the tip of the condom. It does not have to be a hurried affair. You can take your time putting on the condom, playing with the penis as you do so. The more imaginative might like to experiment with ways of getting the condom on to the penis without using their hands. It is important to make sure the condom goes on to the penis once it is erect and before any genital contact occurs to avoid any risk from pre-cum. Immediately after ejaculation the condom-covered penis should be withdrawn, holding the condom on the still-erect penis with the fingers. You can then dispose of the condom in the same way as any other rubbish, in the bin, or down the toilet (but you will need to wrap it in toilet paper to make it flush away).

DOES AND DON'T FOR CONDOM USERS:

Do
- Carry a selection of condoms with you (be prepared)
- Use each condom only once
- Check the date of expiry on the condom packet – *if it has not got one do not use it*
- Use only water-based lubricants
- Use plenty of lubrication
- Expel the air from the condom before unrolling it
- Check that you are unrolling it the right way
- Think about condoms as a challenge and enjoy them!

Safer Sexual Intercourse?

Don't
- Unroll the condom before using it
- Leave them lying around in direct sunlight

WHEN CONDOMS DO NOT WORK

Condoms do not work because: *they're not used* or *they're not used properly*.

Let us look at the first of these. You might decide not to use condoms for a variety of reasons. For instance, you might think that *this* partner could not be infected; he/she refuses to agree to them; you have left them in the car glove compartment; you are afraid to raise the subject; you are too drunk to care.

All of these can and do happen, but they seem to betray a lack of commitment to making condoms part of your sex life. For example the assumption that any partner 'isn't the kind of person who has an infection' is positively dangerous. Partners who will not agree to condoms may be indicating their level of respect for your wishes. If you are really committed to using condoms, you will not be leaving them anywhere, you will always have them handy!

The most common reason for condom failure is misuse: either the condom gets damaged through mishandling resulting in a leak; or else it is put on or taken off incorrectly resulting in seepage. The best way to prevent this happening is to practise and make sure that you know how to use them properly.

CONDOMS: RAISING THE ISSUE WITH YOUR PARTNER

The one question which is often asked about condoms (after the practical details) is how do you persuade partners to agree to them? There is no easy answer to this one. However, having read the sections on communication and assertion you will be aware that one of the important principles in dealing with conflict is being responsible for yourself. For instance, if you are trying to convince a partner to use condoms on the grounds that you are somehow worried about what they might 'give' you, you will probably be less successful than if you present the issue as something you would do with anyone. 'I have a rule for myself about condoms' (see chapter X) is about as non-accusing as you can get. Additionally being positive about the benefits of condoms might help; for example, explaining that they will protect both of you, and emphasizing that you can have a lot of fun with them, or play with them in ways other than their intended use, might help to relax you both.

In the final analysis, however, there is always the possibility that a partner might simply refuse outright. In this event you have some choices to make. You might negotiate other ways of being sexual together that do not require using condoms (see Chapter 8). Or you might decide that the refusal to agree to your wishes makes him/her less appealing as a partner and you would rather not be sexual at all with them.

However, there is also the choice of allowing their dislike of condoms to take precedence over your need for protection and to go ahead with unsafe sex. Only you can decide for yourself if there might be a price for doing so, and if that price is worth paying.

8

Towards Safer Sex

In Chapter 7 we used as a working definition of sexual intercourse 'penetrative sex involving the insertion of the penis into the vagina or anus'. In this chapter we are going to examine some of the definitions we use a little more closely.

The dictionary defines 'intercourse' as 'social communication between individuals'. So we might be justified in expecting sexual intercourse to be defined as 'sexual communication between individuals'. But sexual intercourse is defined as 'insertion of man's penis into woman's vagina'. As we said in Chapter 7 we seem to attach less value to those ways of being sexual that do not involve penetration.

HIV has presented us with both a threat and a challenge. We are continually hearing about this *threat* to our health. Yet we seldom hear about the *challenge*. Indeed we could be forgiven for thinking, if our only source of information has been government leaflets, television, and newspaper advertisements, that safer sex means no sex, less sex, fewer partners, or simply using condoms.

Safer Sex

Safer sex might mean much more than this if we let it. It might mean giving ourselves the chance to explore and value as sexual a whole range of experiences we have hitherto neglected or ignored on the grounds that they were not 'real' sex. Like so much else in life, sex is what you make it.

Also in Chapter 7 we talked a lot about sexual intercourse and how you might go about making it safer. The discussion was specifically addressed to those for whom intercourse was an essential part of their sex lives. However, we are aware that this is not the case for everyone. Even if we apply the relatively simple safety measures we described in Chapter 7, intercourse is still potentially a risky activity. This is not to advise against it, but simply to recommend considering some of the options we describe in this chapter of which you might have been unaware. Many people realize that there are an infinite number of ways of being sexual alone or with a partner that do not include intercourse, and this chapter is both for them and anyone else who is interested in considering some safer sexual alternatives.

One of the safer sex campaigns in the States summed up the safer sex message succinctly in the phrase 'on me not in me'. The message here essentially was that provided the sex you had was non-penetrative (especially penis in vagina or anus) then the sexual world is your erotic oyster! However, the sexual worlds we inhabit reflect our social values. In earlier chapters we talked about the influences that shape the nature, extent and limits of our sexual experiences. Our society is very ambivalent about sex. On the one hand, as we have described, we are bombarded with sexual imagery, yet on the other comes the message that sex is dirty and only for marriage. No wonder many of us are confused!

It is difficult to feel good about *safer* sex if we feel

uncomfortable with *any* sex. If deep down we are uncomfortable with our sexual selves, we are perhaps more likely to behave in ways which reflect such discomfort possibly resulting in unnecessary risk-taking.

It is sometimes said that safer sex takes the spontaneity out of sex and hence ruins it. Even if this *were* the case it certainly does not have to be this way. Perhaps one difficulty about safer sex is that it means that we can no longer avoid talking about sex. If we are really committed to safer sex, we need to discuss this with partners, telling them what we might like to do, and listening to their suggestions and negotiating what sex with them might mean. This is why part of this book has concerned itself with communication skills, because we need these now more than ever.

The good thing about all of this is that apart from making the sex we have safer, we might also make it *better*. Being able to ask for what we want, say 'no' to experiences we do not want and become responsible for ourselves, have always been good ideas when it comes to sex, long before anyone even thought of safer sex.

The sensual–sexual spectrum

The ladder concept we introduced earlier in this book (page 40) illustrated the idea that sexual activity is not a question of an inevitable progression from rung one to rung five, from holding hands to orgasm. Instead it is a spectrum of experience ranging from the subtly sensual to the sublimely sexual – what could be generally described as the erotic.

We have learned to focus most of our attention on the more explicitly sexual feelings at rungs four, five and six. We will talk about these feelings in relation to safer sex a little later, but we would like to concentrate for the time being on those sometimes sensual, sometimes sexual feelings from rungs one to three.

TOUCH

Anyone who has read about or experienced sex therapy will be familiar with 'sensate focus'. Essentially this is about taking people back to rung one and two feelings and encouraging them to explore these, free from the demands of intercourse or orgasm. People are invited to make some time free from interruptions, and in a warm comfortable room, with a relaxing atmosphere, to take turns giving and receiving sensual touching. The emphasis is on being able to do this without becoming preoccupied with what your partner is experiencing. Their responsibility to communicate any discomfort is clearly spelled out to them before they embark on the exercise. The emphasis is also very much on increasing awareness of the sense of touch.

Many of the 'safer sex guidelines' available suggest massage as one way of being safely sexual. However, while we would wholeheartedly endorse this suggestion, we would also recommend that you see it as simply a beginning of safer sexuality. In addition to the sensuality of human skin, there are a variety of other textures which people find exciting or relaxing to touch.

The sense of touch is an extremely important one in sensuality and sexuality. However we have four other senses that we can call upon to help us make sex safer. Let us look at each of these in turn.

SMELL

As humans we seem to have got out of touch with our sense of smell. Not that we ignore it, but rather we seem somewhat uncomfortable with it. We use perfumes and oils to attract partners, but also to cover up our normal body smells. We have an entire industry devoted to disguising vaginal odours, encouraging women to believe that their genital area is somehow a dirty and smelly place. Apart from the effects of this upon women's self-image, the chemicals in these products can interfere with the normal balance of the vagina and lead to problems. This is not to say that the smell of body odour is necessarily pleasant (although it is to some people), but rather that natural body smells can be intensely erotic. Different parts of the body have different smells. Other cultures have appreciated this and designed ways of emphasizing rather than hiding these natural smells. There is now a growing interest among scientists in the role played by 'pheromones' in human sexual behaviour. These are odours, which in some species of animals act as sexual signals, but their role in human sexuality is as yet unclear.

TASTE

The mouth and tongue are exquisitely sensitive organs. Kissing is the most obvious example of the way in which we use our sense of taste in sex, and this seems to be a very important part of most people's sexual lives. Oral sex is another example of the importance of the sense of taste; this may be kissing or licking the genitals of your partner, or else it may be more general body kissing or licking. Apart from the natural body tastes, people create their own sexual tastes by imaginative use of tasty items like yoghurt, or for some, champagne.

SIGHT

The advertising industry thrives on the creative and powerful use of visual imagery. 'Lights off and under-the-blanket sex' excludes the erotic use of the sense of sight. We often forget how important a part it plays in our sexual lives, from admiring and enjoying looking at our own bodies to the assessment of others as to whether we find them attractive or not. There is often no more powerful aphrodisiac in a sexual relationship than looking at and visually enjoying your partner's body. The use of visual erotic material, be it literature, magazines or videos, can be very erotic.

HEARING

Those who subscribe to the myth that you should not have to talk during sex may well not be using one of their senses to the full, thus depriving themselves of another source of erotic stimulation. Listening to your own and your partner's sounds of delight can enhance your pleasure. Background music can be a powerful erotic stimulus. Similarly talking to each other about what you like and enjoy can be a real turn on. 'Talking dirty' can add a sparkle to a fading sexual intensity.

Feelings

Throughout this book we have emphasized the importance of feelings, recognizing, accepting, and dealing with them. Feelings play an essential part in sex; if they are positive, they are what make sex exciting and enjoyable; but if they are negative they can ruin the best of sexual relationships when left unsaid or unresolved. You might be wondering what feelings have got to do with safer sex, but just think about it ... the feeling of anticipation, *knowing* that you are finally going to have sex with that person you have been desiring can be intensely erotic (sometimes better than the reality when it happens) and it is entirely safe. This is not to say that from now on you have to be satisfied simply with thinking about sex, but simply to encourage you to savour and enjoy the feelings you have that contribute to making sex exciting. Feeling close, loved, excited, sexy, are all entirely safe. It is how we act on the basis of what we feel that determines the relative safety of what we are doing.

We are not so naive as to say that safer sex is about not acting on feelings. What we are saying is that it is important to be clear about what feelings you are acting on and why. For instance, using sex as a way of dealing with difficult negative feelings may not be very wise. Sex that comes from anger, resentment or fear, might well turn out to be at your partner's expense, or your own. Even when it does not, you are likely, when it is over, to be left with the same feeling you had when you began.

Making it safer

So how do you put it all together? This, inevitably is up to you. Safer sex is about using the most important sex organ we have ... our brains. If we can deal with our sexual fears and anxieties we can let our brains take over devising ways of making sex safer.

For instance, reading over the previous sections on the senses, you may well have recognized that you have a preference for making use of and enjoying a particular sense. You can then use this information, using your brain in two ways. First, you can begin thinking about other ways that you might develop that sense in imaginative ways. For instance, if you are primarily a visual person and enjoy looking at your partner, you might like to think a little more carefully about how you might enhance this sense. For example you could wear clothes you find particularly erotic, or ask your partner to do so, agreeing that you will do something to help them develop his/her favourite sense in return. Who would have thought negotiation could be so much fun?

Second, you might like to develop those senses you tend to use less or even ignore. So using the example above, if you are primarily a visual person, you might try wearing a blindfold the next time you are in a sexual situation and concentrate on your sense of smell, taste or touch. If you are primarily a tactile person you might decide to make a list of ways you might have sex without touching your partner.

Fantasy

Fantasy is an integral part of human life, and erotic or sexual fantasy is an important part of sexual life. Nancy Friday, who has researched the field of human sexual fantasy, says it should be thought of as an extension of one's sexual life. When fantasies are positive and pleasurable, they can enrich our erotic lives; when they are negative and frightening they can seriously interfere with our sexual pleasure. Fantasy can be a way of being sexually omnipotent. We can be successful, attractive, and most important get exactly the kind of pleasure we desire. Fantasies can be elaborate, detailed imaginary sequences of events, or else they can be sudden, fleeting glimpses of images we find sexually exciting or interesting. Fantasy can be a substitute for sex, it can lead to sex,

Towards Safer Sex

it can bring additional pleasure to sex, and it can be simply an end in itself.

Kinsey, the famous researcher, found that most men and women fantasize when they masturbate, and that many do so when they are having sex with a partner. This often causes difficulty for some people, who feel guilty for what they see as 'betrayal' of their partner. On the other hand there are those who feel guilty not for having fantasies, but for what those fantasies consist of. The fact that people have sexual fantasies does not mean that they will act them out. Indeed part of the joy of sexual fantasy is that it is, if we want it to be, the most private aspect of our sexual lives. We can give free reign to thoughts and imagery we would neither wish nor be able to act out in reality.

Safer sex: putting it all together

In this chapter we have introduced what we think are the basic ingredients of safer sex. It is now up to you to take these and concoct your own recipes based on your own particular tastes and preferences.

If you have agreed with a partner that you are going to have safer sex together then you are already halfway there. All you need to do now is to decide what that is going to mean in practical terms. If you do not have a regular partner, or the partner you have is resistant to the idea of introducing safer sex into your relationship, you might like to concentrate on Chapter 6 with its emphasis on communication skills. You might also like to do some of the exercises we offer towards the end of this chapter which may help you to use your imagination to construct safer sexual activities that will appeal to both of you.

Safer Sex

What you could do is to agree that you will experiment with safer sex for a trial period and then at the end of that period assess how you feel about it, paying particular attention to the positives you have gained from the experience.

DEVELOPING THE SENSES

Read that section of this chapter again and think about which senses you use and enjoy most during sex, and those you might like to use more. It is best to be realistic, so attempt to devise three ways in which you could enhance your enjoyment of a sense you do not normally pay much attention to. Then when you have done this do the same with the next one, and so on until you have experimented with all of your senses. If you have a partner you can offer each other suggestions and learn from each other's experience and preferences. Remember to be as creative as possible. So if you wanted to experiment with the sense of taste, you might for instance try drinking wine or champagne from your partner's navel. Or else if you wanted to experiment with your visual sense you might like to buy some erotic literature or magazines to whet your sexual appetite.

DEVELOPING YOUR FANTASY LIFE

Many of us have favourite fantasies. Begin by thinking what these are for you. Before immersing yourself into that fantasy think about the senses, and in turn go through the fantasy concentrating on one sense at a time. Think about what part that sense plays in your fantasy. If you find that you simply do not use some of your senses in your fantasy think about how you might include that particular sensual awareness.

Towards Safer Sex

When you have done this you could begin concentrating more specifically on the content of your fantasies. There are now several books available which deal with sexual fantasies (see Appendix 3). Some of these describe common (and uncommon) themes in sexual fantasy and you might find these give you both permission to continue fantasizing, as well as some impetus to develop your own existing fantasy life or to create some new ones.

Some people enjoy acting out their fantasies in a limited way. If this appeals to you, then you might decide together with your partner that you will help each other to make this possible, provided of course that such activity is both safe and acceptable to both partners. Additionally you will need to agree to treat such personal sharing with the respect which it deserves! If you are likely to find listening to your partner's fantasies distressing, threatening or jealousy-provoking – do not do it. Fantasies can be dramatic, irrational, bizarre, funny and most of all very powerful. It is important to recognize that they are *fantasies* not reality.

Finally you might also like to keep a diary of your own fantasies to provide you with some erotic pleasure or stimulation when you want it. You can keep this entirely private or you might agree with a partner to exchange excerpts from your diaries!

Devising safer sexual activities

First, think back over your sexual life and write down all the most erotic, sensual and sexual experiences you have ever had or wanted to have. Give yourself plenty of time to do this and make your list as full and as detailed as possible. When you have done this go through your list and assess these events in terms of their safety (following the 'on me not in me' guideline). You can either delete those activities that are (were) unsafe, or modify them to make them safer. So for instance if one of your most sensual activities was 'fucking in the back of a car', you could modify it either to include using a condom, or else to include non-penetrative sex. When you have done this what you will be left with is a list of safer sexual alternatives that have been important to you at one time or another in your sexual life. You can then use this as the basis for expanding and developing other ideas.

Second, either alone or with a partner you might like to simply write down any and every erotic idea or image you have that could come under the following headings:

massage · dressing-up · undressing · baths/showers · masturbation · kissing · sucking · underwear · hair · fruit · blue movies · erotic literature · jacuzzis · saunas · different venues · voyeurism · sex without touching · sex using only your mouth · creative ways of using condoms · erotic noises · rubbing · role-playing · sensual oils · using food · posing · mirrors · toes and feet · armpits · bondage · telephone calls · sex toys

Again, when you have done this you can go through these ideas and amend or delete for safety reasons. What you are left with should be a huge range of safer sexual options. You can then swap lists and see how imaginative each of you is. You can then turn theory into practice by agreeing to take turns experimenting with ideas from each other's lists, again the only conditions being that they are both safe and acceptable.

Finishing off safely

We have talked a lot about the lower levels of sensual and sexual excitement. However, for most people sex is usually related to orgasm. Since orgasm for men is generally linked to ejaculation, and since in terms of HIV semen is potentially very dangerous as a means of virus transmission, we need to look at how we can enjoy orgasm in safety.

FOR MEN

Men usually have four options for the means they use to come: first, they can masturbate or be masturbated to orgasm; second, they can be on the receiving end of oral sex; third, they can climax inside their partner; finally (and rarely) they can come purely from the power of their most powerful sex organ ... no, not the one between their legs, but the one between their ears! Obviously ejaculating on to your partner, or in midair is no problem. However, doing so inside your partner may be problematic from the point of view of safety. Withdrawal before ejaculation occurs is still risky because of pre-cum. So unless you are using a condom the message from your partner may be 'on me not in me'. You might feel cheated by being informed that coming inside your partner is no longer such a wise idea; however, it is important to be aware that at least one major sex survey has reported that many men find the orgasms they have from either masturbating themselves, or being masturbated by a partner, are more intense than those they have during intercourse.

Safer Sex

> **EXERCISE**
> This one is aimed at men. Write down as many ways as you can think of to have your orgasm, remembering the maxim 'on me not in me'. If you are having difficulty being imaginative you might like to ask your partner to help. Then you can turn from theory into practice.

FOR WOMEN

From a safety point of view, orgasm for women is simply not a problem, unless of course you prefer or can only come when you are having intercourse. If this is the case, there are two more options. You can decide that you want to continue having intercourse, and make sure your partner uses a condom. Or else you might like to try a little help from a (mechanical) friend.

THE VIBRATOR

Vibrators are essentially hand-held battery or mains operated devices which vibrate, and when placed next to the skin stimulate the nerves to produce a usually pleasant sensation. According to the surveys we mentioned earlier in this book, they are very popular; one in eight of the women in one survey owned one, and four out of ten reported using them.

Women may like to apply the vibrator directly to the clitoris and the surrounding area, while men report pleasurable sensation when it is applied to the glans of the penis or the perineum, the area between the testicles and the anus.

If you are thinking about buying one it is wise to shop around. Some come with adjustable speeds and attachments. You can only insert the battery-operated models into the vagina or rectum, but be very careful with the latter, as vibrators can slip inside and cause serious damage.

The vibrator, apart from helping numerous women (and men) to reach orgasm has numerous sensual and sexual uses for the adventurous. Apart from the range of phallic-shaped objects available in sex shops, a range of battery-operated personal massagers is available from large chemist shops. If looked after properly and kept away from water these are perfectly safe.

Sex shops

You might consider a tour of some sex shops investigating the range of sexual accoutrements that are available these days. Because sex shops have traditionally been male territory, and are designed to whet the sexual appetites of men, some women feel uncomfortable at the thought of visiting one. Going with a friend might help relieve your discomfort. However you should not leave either your commonsense or your values at home. We are not saying that you will, or ought, to find what you see acceptable personally or politically. You may find some of what you see interesting, amusing, boring or degrading.

You will find vibrators shaped like penises in a range of sizes (small, medium and liar!), clitoral stimulators, a dazzling array of various types of condoms, dildoes, underwear, magazines, videos and a range of pills, sprays and creams all claiming to turn us from the sexually inadequate into the sexually superhuman. Some people find sex shops morally offensive while others will find them a source of inspiration and fun.

Safer Sex

Practical suggestions

We hope that by now, having read this book, you will have understood the concepts of safer sex. However you may be saying to yourself 'this is all fine in theory, but what about the practice?' To set you on your way we offer you some ideas. From here on it is up to you!

LOOK, NO HANDS

Whether you are having intercourse or not, condoms can (if you let them) be fun. See if you can get a condom on to your partner without using your hands!

SEX GAMES

What about introducing some safer sexual games into your relationships? Forfeits, strip poker, and all those other card games can take on a new life in the light of safer sex.

TO THE BRINK AND BACK AGAIN

Tease your partner. Get him/her to the brink and then not let them come! And again, and again, until *you* are ready! This will sharpen up your negotiation skills too.

HANGIN' ON THE TELEPHONE

What about using those telephone extensions creatively? You can talk to each other as if you were miles apart about what you would like to do, then 'lo and behold' he/she walks into the room!

SHOWING OFF YOUR COLLECTION

Why not keep a record of your favourite sexual fantasies? These can be of your own (or other people's) creation and will be a useful stimulus to use when you are alone. Or when you want to excite each other you can swap records! You can add to this over the years. You might find it interesting or amusing to look back on it some day!

DRESSING-DOWN

How about keeping your clothes on for as long as possible? You might find that you do not manage to get completely naked! This might also help you see *DRESSING-UP* in a completely new light!

These are just suggestions – the rest, as ever, is up to you!

CONCLUSION

A Way Forward

Life is full of risks. We hope that this book has offered you a chance to reconsider some of the risks in *your* life particularly in relation to sexuality. You may not find answers – there may not be any – but you may find ways to feel more comfortable living with uncertainty.

AIDS sums up many of the uncertainties of the world in which we live: all the issues we try to avoid because of the difficult feelings they evoke. Sadly it seems that AIDS and HIV infection will be linked to sexuality for the foreseeable future. While it may mean the end of 'carefree' sex (if there ever was such a thing), it does not mean the end of sexual pleasure. Far from it. AIDS presents us with some basic challenges about the way we live our lives and express our sexuality. If we can face up to these challenges, we may find ourselves enriched by the experience. We do not pretend it will be easy, but as a society we have never been very much at ease with sexuality, so what have we got to lose?

At the most basic level we are now being presented with an opportunity to confront our fears and to learn

A Way Forward

to live our sexual lives with responsibility, care and respect for ourselves and others. If we can do this, we might just find that *safer sex* might also be *better* sex. Instead of being a loss or denial of our sexuality, safer sex might turn out to be a celebration of it, of our relationships and of sex itself.

APPENDIX 1

Useful Organizations

We have tried to make these lists as accurate and reliable as possible, however things change very quickly. If in doubt clarify the information with one of the well known switchboards or hotlines.

United Kingdom

Terence Higgins Trust
BM AIDS
London WC1 3XX
tel: 01 240 1010
National AIDS Helpline
tel: 0800 567 123
London Lesbian and Gay Switchboard
tel: 01 837 7324
Body Positive
PO Box 493
London W14 0TF
tel: 01 373 9124

Family Planning Association
27-35 Mortimer Street
London W1N 7RJ
tel: 01 636 7866
Welsh AIDS Campaign
PO Box 348
Cardiff CF1 4XL
tel: 0222 223443
Scottish AIDS Monitor
PO Box 169
Edinburgh EH1 3UU
tel: 031 558 1167
Standing Conference On Drug Abuse
1 Hatton Place
London EC1
tel: 01 430 2341

Useful Organizations

Australia

Sydney AIDS Hotline
02 332 4000
*AIDS Council of
New South Wales*
PO Box 350
Darlinghurst
New South Wales - 2010
Bobbi Goldsmith Foundation
PO Box 97
Darlinghurst
New South Wales - 2010
Ankali Project
(support for people with HIV infection)
tel: 332 4000

Canada

AIDS Community of Toronto
PO Box 55
Station F
Toronto N4Y 2LH
tel: 926 1626

France

AIDES
BP 759
75123 Paris
Cedex 03
tel: 01 4272 1999

Italy

AIECS
Rome
tel: 859 642

Japan

AIDS Hotline
Tokyo
tel: 823 2101

Netherlands

National AIDS Information Line
tel: 06 321 2120

Switzerland

AHS (AIDS information and support)
23 - 6786
Postfach 7660 8023
Zurich
tel: 23 6786

United States of America

Gay Men's Health Crisis
Box 274
132 West 24th St
New York
NY 10011
tel: (212) 807 7035/6664
Boston AIDS Action Committee
661 Boyleston St
Boston
Mass
MA 02116
tel: (617) 437 6200

Safer Sex

San Francisco AIDS Foundation
333 Valencia St
San Francisco
CA 94103
tel: 863 AIDS

West Germany

Deutch AIDS Hilfe
Niebuhrstrasse 71
1000 Berlin
12
tel: 860 651

APPENDIX 2

Useful Addresses in the United Kingdom

Abortion: help, information and support

British Pregnancy Advisory Service, Head Office, Austy Manor, Wootten Wawen, Solihull, West Midlands B95 6BX (tel: 0564 23225)

Pregnancy Advisory Service, 11–13 Charlotte Street, London W1P 1HD (tel: 01 637 8962)

Alcohol and drug abuse

Accept National Services, 200 Seagrove Road, London SW6 1RQ (tel: 01 381 3155)

Alcohol Counselling Service, 34 Electric Lane, London SW9 (tel: 01 737 3579/0)

Release, 169 Commercial Street, London E1 6BW (tel: 01 377 5905) Legal advice and counselling on drugs

Women's Alcohol Centre, 254 St Paul's Road, London N1 2LJ (tel: 01 226 4581)

Assertion courses

Adult Education Institutes: check local libraries, local telephone directories

Family Planning Association, Education Unit, 27–31 Mortimer St, London W1 (tel: 01 636 7866)

Women's Centres, for addresses contact: A Woman's Place (tel: 01 930 0715)

Women's Therapy Centre, 6 Manor Gardens, London N7 6LA (tel: 01 263 6200)

Bookshops

A few London bookshops with a wide range of books on sexuality and personal relationships:

Compendium Bookshop, 234 Camden High Street, London NW1 (tel: 01 485 8944)

Family Planning Association Bookshop, 27 Mortimer St, London W1N 7RJ (tel: 01 636 7866)

Gay's the Word Bookshop, 66 Marchmont Street, London WC1 (tel: 01 278 7654)

Silver Moon Women's Bookshop, 68 Charing Cross Rd, London WC2 (tel: 01 836 7906)

Sister Write Bookshop and Gallery, 190 Upper Street, London N1 (tel: 01 226 9782)

Contraception

Brook Advisory Centres: counselling and advice for young people 153A East Street, London SE17 2SD (tel: 01 708 1234)

Family Planning Association: advice and information service on birth control and reproductive health, 27–35 Mortimer Street, London W1N 7RJ (tel: 01 636 7866)

Marie Stopes House: contraception/abortion/counselling/well woman clinic, 108 Whitfield Street, London W1 (tel: 01 388 0662/2585)

Useful Addresses in the United Kingdom

Eating problems

Anorexia and Bulimia Nervosa Association – ABNA confidential phone line run by women: Tottenham Women and Health Centre, Annexe C, London N15 4RX (tel: 01 885 3936, helpline Wednesdays 6–9 pm)

Anorexic Aid, The Priory Centre, 11 Priory Rd, High Wycombe, Bucks HP13 6SL (tel: 0494 21431)

Fat Women's Group: support group challenging negative stereotypes and prejudice against fat women, c/o WRRIC, 52–54 Featherstone Street, London EC1H 8RT (tel: 01 806 7096)

Overeaters Anonymous: mixed groups in Britain and Ireland, c/o Manor Gardens Centre, 6–9 Manor Gardens, London N7 (tel: 01 868 4109)

Health

Breast Care and Mastectomy Association: practical and emotional support for women, 26 Harrison St, London WC1H 8JG (tel: 01 837 0908)

DAWN (Drugs, Alcohol, Women, Nationally), Omnibus Workspace, 39–41 North Road, London N7 9DP (tel: 01 700 4653)

Health Education Authority Resources Centre, 78 New Oxford Street London WC1A 1AH (tel: 01 631 0930)

Herpes Association, 41 North Road, London N7 9DP (tel: 01 609 9061, helpline)

The Haemophilia Society, 123 Westminster Bridge Road, London SE1 7HR (tel: 01 928 2020)

London Lesbian and Gay Switchboard: (tel: 01 837 7324)

Terrence Higgins Trust: counselling, information, welfare, legal advice to people regarding AIDS and related conditions

Daily helpline, tel: 01 242 1010 (3–10 pm)

Safer Sex

Women's Health Information Centre: library and resource centre including well woman clinics, 52–54 Featherstone Street, London EC1Y 8RT (tel: 01 251 6580)

Women's National Cancer Control Campaign, 1 South Audley Street, London W1Y 5DQ (tel: 01 499 7532/4)

Therapy and Workshops

(Including personal/sexual counselling and sexuality groups)

Association of Sex and Marital Therapists, P.O. Box 62, Sheffield S10 3TS

British Association for Counselling, 37a Sheep Street, Rugby CV21 3BX (tel: 0788 78328)

Help Advisory Centre, 3 Adam and Eve Mews, London W8 (tel: 01 937 7687/6445)

Identity, 2 Warwick Crescent, London W2 (tel: 01 289 6175)

London Lesbian and Gay Switchboard (tel: 01 837 7324)

New Grapevine, 416 St John Street, London WC1 (tel: office 01 278 9157, helpline 01 278 9147)

PACE (Project for Advice, Counselling and Education) c/o London Lesbian and Gay Centre, 67/9 Cowcross Street, London EC1 (tel: 01 251 2689)

Pellin Feminist Therapy Centre, 43 Killyon Rd, London SW8 2XS (tel: 01 622 0148)

Relate (formerly Marriage Guidance Council), National Office, Herbert Gray College, Little Church Street, Rugby CV21 3AP (tel: 0788 73241)

Spectrum, 49 Croftdown Road, London NW5 1EL (tel: 01 485 5259)

Women's Therapy Centre, 6 Manor Gardens, London N7 6LA (tel: 01 263 6200)

APPENDIX 3: Further Reading

HIV and AIDS

Altman, D., *AIDS and the New Puritanism*, Pluto Press, 1986

National Institute of Medicine and National Academy of Sciences, *Mobilizing Against AIDS: The Unfinished Story*, Harvard University Press, 1986

Panos Institute, *AIDS and the Third World*, Panos Institute, Revised 1987

Patton C., *Making It: A Woman's Guide to Sex in the Age of AIDS*, Firebrand Press, 1987

Patton C., *Sex and Germs: The Politics of AIDS*, South End Press, 1985

Chirimuuta R.C. & R.J., *AIDS Africa and Racism*, Burton on Trent: 1987

Peabody B., *The Screaming Room*, Oak Tree Publications, 1986

Vass A., *A Plague in US*, Venus Academica, 1986

Tatchell P., *AIDS: A Guide to Survival*, Gay Men's Press, 1986 (revised 1987)

Frontliners, *Living with AIDS: A Guide to Survival by People with AIDS*, Frontliners, 1987

Safer Sex

It is difficult to keep up to date with information about HIV and AIDS. The following magazines are useful regular sources of information:

New Scientist
Capital Gay
Scientific American
Nature
The Economist

Assertion and communication skills

Berne, Eric, *Games People Play*, Penguin, 1968
Butler, Pamela, *Self-Assertion for Women*, Harper and Row, 1976
Dickson, Anne, *A Woman in Your Own Right – Assertiveness and You*, Quartet, 1982
Smith, Manuel, *When I Say No, I Feel Guilty*, Dial, 1975

Health

Adler, M.W., *ABC of Sexually Transmitted Diseases*, British Medical Association, 1984
Miller, David, *Living with HIV*, Macmillan, 1987
Phillips, Angela and Rakusen, Jill, *Our Bodies Ourselves*, Penguin, 1978. Excellent sections on breast and genital examination for women
Zilbergeld, Bernard, *Men and Sex*, Fontana, 1980

Massage and touching

Downing, G. *The Massage Book*, Penguin, 1977
Masters, W. and Johnson, V., *The Pleasure Bond*, Little, Brown, 1974
Montagu, Ashley, *Touching*, Perennial Library, 1971

Sexuality

Brown, Paul and Faulder, Caroline, *Treat Yourself to Sex*, Penguin, 1979

Dickson, Anne *The Mirror Within – A New Look at Sexuality*, Quartet, 1985

Dodgson, Betty, *Liberating Masturbation*, New York, 1975

Everyman, Oxford University Press, 1982

Friday, Nancy, *My Secret Garden*, Quartet, 1973

Heiman, Julia, Lo Piccolo, Lesley and Lo Piccolo, Joseph *Becoming Orgasmic: A Sexual Growth Program for Women*, Prentice Hall, 1976

Hite, Shere, *The Hite Report*, Dell, 1976; *Women and Love*, Viking 1988

Hooper, Ann, *The Body Electric*, Virago, 1980

Metcalfe, Andy and Humphries, Martin, *Sexuality of Men*, Pluto Press, 1985

Meulenbelt, Anja, *For Ourselves*, Sheba, 1981

Phillips, Angela and Rakusen, Jill, *Our Bodies Ourselves*, Penguin, 1978

Vance, C. (ed.), *Pleasure and Danger*, Routledge and Kegan Paul, 1984

Weeks, J., *Sexuality*, Ellis Horwood Ltd of Tavistock Publications, 1986

Zilbergeld, Bernard, *Men and Sex*, Fontana, 1980

Index

acquired immune deficiency
 syndrome,
 (AIDS), 1, 11, 126
 see also HIV; STD
aggressiveness and
 assertiveness, 79–81
alcohol and sex, 3–4, 89
anal intercourse, 96–7, 103
assertion skills, 6, 23, 28–9,
 79–81, 89–90

body inventory, 45–7
body language, 79
breasts, 7–8, 84

cancer
 breast, 7–8
 cervical, 1, 7, 13–15, 99
celibacy, 25, 54–8
 myths about, 56–7
cervical cancer, 1, 7, 13–15,
 99

 smear test, 14–15
clitoral stimulation, 38, 65,
 67, 96, 123
cock rings, 69, 104
communication skills, 28–9,
 41, 72, 75–83
 see also words
condoms, 14, 89–91, 98–108,
 123–4
 dual role of, 99–100
 failure, 100, 107
 standards of, 103–4
contraception, 99
 barrier methods, 14, 100
 condoms, 14, 89–91,
  98–104
 oral, 5, 13
cuddling, 40, 41

diet and health, 3
dressing up/dressing down,
 125

drugs and sex, 4–5, 89

education, sex, 20–1, 34–5
exercise
  pelvic muscle, 8–9
  physical and stress, 6

family influences and sexual attitudes, 31–2
fantasy, sexual, 64, 70, 116–17, 118–19
feelings, 77–9, 88, 114–15
foreplay, 97
frenulum, 68

gender roles, 31, 33–5, 123
genitals
  care of, 7
  self-examination of, 7–8, 48–50
  words describing, 84

herpes virus, 13, 99
human immunodeficiency virus (HIV), 109
  antibody test, 11–12, 16
  infection, 1–2, 126
  transmission of, 10, 99
  see also AIDS; STD
human papilloma virus (HPV), 13

'I' language, 76, 78, 80, 108
imagination and sex, 64, 124–5
  see also fantasy
intercourse, 44, 85, 109
  anal, 96–7, 103
  as 'full' sex, 21–4, 33, 34, 37–8, 96
  oral, 12, 85, 102
  role in sexual life, 94–8, 110

kissing, 113
KY jelly, 102, 106

ladder concept, 39–43, 111–12

massage, 112
masturbation, 43, 59, 61–2
  female, 62, 65–7
  male, 68–70, 96
  myths about, 31–2, 60–1
  and self-esteem, 70–1
  words describing, 84
media and sexuality, 35–7, 110
monogamy, 24, 33, 92
myths about sex/sexuality, 31–2, 54–8, 60–1, 114

non-oxinol 9, 103

'on me not in me', 110, 120–2
oral
  contraceptives, 5, 13
  sex, 12, 85, 102, 113
orgasm
  in men, 96, 121–2
  simultaneous, 38–9
  in women, 38, 42, 96, 122

pelvic muscle exercise, 8–9
penetrative sex *see*

intercourse
pheromones, 113
pornography, 20

religion and sexual attitudes, 33

self-esteem, 72–4
self-examination of breasts and genitals, 7–8, 12–13, 48–50
see also body inventory
self-pleasuring, 51–3, 63–71
see also masturbation
sensate focus, 112
senses and sexual pleasure, 32, 65–6, 68–9, 112–16, 118
serial monogamy, 92
sex/sexual
anal, 96–7, 103
communication, 86–8
education, 20–1, 34–5
fantasy, 64, 70, 116–19
language, 83–5
myths about, 31–2, 54–8, 60–1, 114
oral, 12, 85, 102, 113
pleasure, ladder of, 39–43, 111–12
'revolution' of the 1960s, 18–19, 21
roles, 31, 33–5, 123
safer, rewards of, 27–9
shops, 123
sexually transmitted disease (STD), 1–2, 9–17
clinics, 12, 15–17
smegma, 7, 13
smoking and health, 4, 13, 14
social pressures and sexual relationships, 22, 32–3, 37, 54
spermicides, 102–3
stress, 5–6

vibrators, 65–7, 69, 122–3

words and sexuality, 50–1, 83–5